I would like to dedicate this book to my Grandmother, who taught me to always have faith.

I want to give special thanks to:

My boys, who gave so much for me to write this book. My husband, Rick, thank you for supporting me as I fulfilled my dream. My sons, Richard, Hunter, and Cobra, thank you for inspiring me and teaching me the value of quality time.

For my 2nd mother, Joyce, thank you for helping so much with my boys. I couldn't have done this without you!

For my mother and father, thank you for being so supportive. Thank you for all you have taught me and given me to be able to accomplish this goal.

For my sisters and brother, all my family and friends, I am so thankful for all your support and faith in me.

For Susan Bastable, thank you for believing in me and giving me my first writing opportunity.

For everyone at Jones and Bartlett, especially Amanda Clerkin, Amy Sibley, Patricia Donnelly, and Rachel Shuster, thank you all for an amazing, educational journey.

JONES AND BARTLETT PUBLISHERS
Sudbury, Massachusetts
BOSTON   TORONTO   LONDON   SINGAPORE

World Headquarters

Jones and Bartlett Publishers
40 Tall Pine Drive
Sudbury, MA 01776
978-443-5000
info@jbpub.com
www.jbpub.com

Jones and Bartlett Publishers
Canada
6339 Ormindale Way
Mississauga, Ontario L5V 1J2
Canada

Jones and Bartlett Publishers
International
Barb House, Barb Mews
London W6 7PA
United Kingdom

Jones and Bartlett's books and products are available through most bookstores and online booksellers. To contact Jones and Bartlett Publishers directly, call 800-832-0034, fax 978-443-8000, or visit our website, www.jbpub.com.

Substantial discounts on bulk quantities of Jones and Bartlett's publications are available to corporations, professional associations, and other qualified organizations. For details and specific discount information, contact the special sales department at Jones and Bartlett via the above contact information or send an email to specialsales@jbpub.com.

The authors, editor, and publisher have made every effort to provide accurate information. However, they are not responsible for errors, omissions, or for any outcomes related to the use of the contents of this book and take no responsibility for the use of the products and procedures described. Treatments and side effects described in this book may not be applicable to all people; likewise, some people may require a dose or experience a side effect that is not described herein. Drugs and medical devices are discussed that may have limited availability controlled by the Food and Drug Administration (FDA) for use only in a research study or clinical trial. Research, clinical practice, and government regulations often change the accepted standard in this field. When consideration is being given to use of any drug in the clinical setting, the health care provider or reader is responsible for determining FDA status of the drug, reading the package insert, and reviewing prescribing information for the most up-to-date recommendations on dose, precautions, and contraindications, and determining the appropriate usage for the product. This is especially important in the case of drugs that are new or seldom used.

Production Credits

Publisher: Kevin Sullivan
Acquisitions Editor: Amy Sibley
Associate Editor: Patricia Donnelly
Editorial Assistant: Rachel Shuster
Production Editor: Amanda Clerkin
Marketing Manager: Rebecca Wasley

V.P., Manufacturing and Inventory Control: Therese Connell
Composition: Auburn Associates, Inc.
Cover and Title Page Design: Kristin E. Parker
Cover and Title Page Image: © Joao Estevao Freitas/Dreamstime.com
Printing and Binding: Malloy, Inc.
Cover Printing: Malloy, Inc.

Library of Congress Cataloging-in-Publication Data
Dart, Michelle A.
    Motivational interviewing in nursing practice : empowering the patient / Michelle A. Dart.
        p. ; cm.
    Includes bibliographical references and index.
    ISBN-13: 978-0-7637-7385-4 (alk. paper)
    ISBN-10: 0-7637-7385-9 (alk. paper)
    1. Nurse and patient. 2. Motivational interviewing. I. Title.
    [DNLM: 1. Counseling—methods. 2. Health Promotion—methods. 3. Motivation. 4. Patient Education as Topic—methods. WY 87 D226m 2011]
    RT86.3.D37 2011
    610.7306'99—dc22
                                            2009038826
6048

Printed in the United States of America
14 13 12   10 9 8 7 6 5 4 3

Table of Contents

Introduction

Nursing, as a profession, is in a unique position to not only accommodate change, but to also help patients endure the path to change. Since nursing began, there have been many changes in how we practice. Initially, nurses were seen primarily as caretakers. Over time, this role has expanded to include roles of educator, counselor, and coach. Nurses educate about health conditions and treatment. As counselors, we help patients to cope with their diagnosis and feelings about their health and well-being. Nurses are also in a role to coach patients to promote behavior change.

With the inception of Healthy People 2000, initiatives were created to help guide our practice to improve the overall health of our country. These initiatives focus on prevention, primarily, but can also be seen as a push to focus on current issues that could lead to improvement in a present health problem or overall health. For this reason there is a need to incorporate coaching into nursing practice. Motivational interviewing is one way to provide this coaching to promote behavior change. With Healthy People still going strong, we are on the cusp of Healthy People 2020. At the time of this writing the Healthy People 2020 goals have not yet been released. It can be concluded from the past initiatives that the goals will include issues surrounding obesity, physical activity, and heart disease, to name just a few (see www.healthypeople.gov). As a result, nurses will need to be better equipped to motivate patients to take charge of their health and well-being.

Motivational interviewing is a method of promoting behavior change through coaching using therapeutic communication. Nurses have learned and often use therapeutic communication in practice. This has been particularly useful in the realm of psychiatric nursing. Motivational interviewing was first created to be used in therapy by psychologists and social workers. Throughout the book this form of communication and model for behavior change is reviewed and its use in nursing practice demonstrated. The nursing profession now has yet another tool to improve how we practice and interact with our patients.

Consider how ritualistic our behaviors become, from the process of showering, the pattern in which we brush our teeth, travel to work or proceed through the grocery store. Now consider the daily habits we succumb to, regardless of the positive or negative impact on our life. Imagine the amount of conscious energy it would take to change one of those rituals. Try it. It is not easy. We, as nurses, need to be equipped to help our patients break through the rituals and improve their health care. Motivational interviewing offers us a way to help patients evaluate their rituals and what it means to release them or cherish them. This book provides techniques to help the patient become more self-aware, as well as increase the nurse's self-awareness. With these and other techniques the nursing profession can excel at promoting behavior change.

In this text, we will explore the many reasons why we would strive for healthier be-haviors. Many statistics are reviewed to demonstrate the state of our nation's health. Self-management skills and insight into health behaviors can promote a desire to be more self-efficacious. As nurses, we cannot change another person's behaviors. What we can do is walk beside our patients as they travel the path toward change.

Basics of Motivational Interviewing

HOW MOTIVATIONAL INTERVIEWING BEGAN

William R. Miller, PhD, published a paper in 1983 entitled "Motivational Interviewing with Problem Drinkers" (Miller, 1996). This was the beginning of a new era. A challenging arena, drug and alcohol counseling took on a new facility for change. Where counselors had struggled to find ways to help people afflicted with addictions, there was now a model to assist the counselor in promoting behavior change. Miller went from this one paper, one in which he had not even intended to publish, to develop the cornerstone for all healthcare providers to promote changes in behavior in patients who struggle with

1

adversities and addictions (Miller, 1996). Miller believed that motivation is not a personality trait but a state of readiness. This state of readiness fluctuates over time and needs to be assessed at each encounter to determine if a patient is ready to move forward with a change in behavior (Britt, Hudson, & Blampied, 2004).

It is not surprising that Miller became motivated himself to research and discover all he could about this practice-changing concept. In 1989 Stephen Rollnick joined Miller in the quest for a model to help shape the practice of promoting behavior change. Together, they worked on formalizing this model they called "**motivational interviewing**" so they could then share their knowledge with others in their field (Miller & Rollnick, 2002).

The ideas were solid, but the needs of their colleagues required them to rethink their teachings. Miller and Rollnick knew that not everyone fully understood motivational interviewing, and they went on to fine tune the motivational interviewing model. Together, they wrote a second edition book to help practitioners better understand the concept that was found to spread across the professions to anyone in the clinical field, including nurses (Miller & Rollnick, 2002). With their tools in our hands, we have begun to use this model in various areas of practice. What was once thought to be useful only in the counseling field, the tactics of motivational interviewing could be used in a variety of populations and not restricted to the realm of addictions.

WHAT MOTIVATIONAL INTERVIEWING IS

There are many words used to describe motivational interviewing. It is found in writings as a brief intervention or negotiation, counseling method, therapeutic communication, and a way of walking or dancing with the patient. By definition, "Motivational Interviewing is a directive, client-centered counseling style for eliciting behavior change by helping clients to explore and resolve **ambivalence**" (Rollnick & Miller, 1995, p. 325). Ambivalence is a state of uncertainty. It is like standing in the middle of a teeter totter and debating on which side to go. One side represents accepting the way things are and not changing a thing, whereas the other side is a place to begin the journey to behavior change.

There is a theoretical basis to motivational interviewing. Because of the scope of this book, the guiding theory is only discussed briefly. The transtheoretical model, created by Carlo DiClemente and James Prochaska, guides motivational interviewing (Miller & Rollnick, 2002). There are other theories that can be explored as to the relationship to motivational interviewing, but this model is chosen to review because of the effectiveness of this model in this framework. Within this model are the five stages of change, reviewed in Figure 1-1 (Kumm, Hicks, Shupe, & Hagemaster, 2002; Lange & Tigges, 2005; Shinitzky & Kub,

2001). These stages of change are part of a cycle. In the maintenance stage reevaluation can occur and the whole cycle can begin again.

The transtheoretical model demonstrates 10 processes of change that promotes advancement through the stages of change. Moving from precontemplation to contemplation and onto preparation stages involves the processes of consciousness raising, dramatic relief, environmental reevaluation, and self-reevaluation. In the preparation stage self-liberation occurs. Moving from these stages to action and maintenance involves the following processes: contingency management, counterconditioning, helping relationships, reinforcement management, and stimulus control (Lange & Tigges, 2005; Shinitzky & Kub, 2001).

Four main principles guide the motivational interviewing technique: **express empathy**, support self-efficacy, **develop discrepancy**, and roll with resistance (Levensky, Forcehimes, O'Donohue, & Beitz, 2007; Rolfe, 2004; Miller, Zweben, DiClemente, & Rychtarik, 1992) (Figure 1-2). As noted in Figure 1-2,

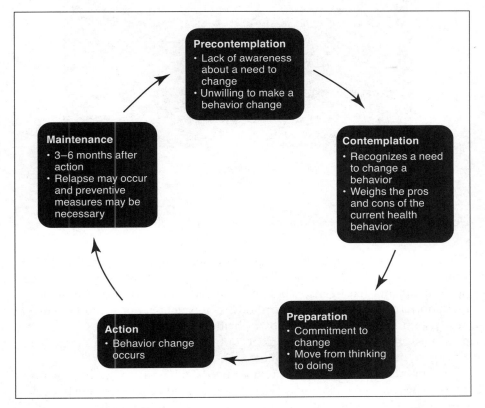

Figure 1-1 Stages of Change

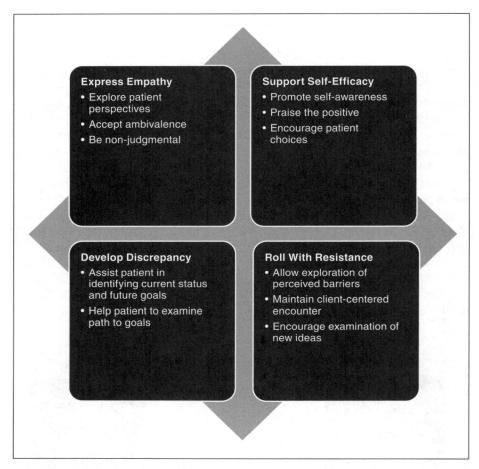

Figure 1-2   Principles of Motivational Interviewing

these four main principles need to be maintained to have a therapeutic inter-action with a patient. Expressing empathy allows the patient to feel comfortable opening up and sharing his or her personal perspectives. It is important to re-main objective and expect a patient to be ambivalent about his or her current health status. The patient is often overwhelmed by a recent diagnosis, frustrated over failed efforts, angry about a lack of control over the situation, or may, in fact, already be motivated to make a change.

To support **self-efficacy** the provider needs to be sure to not impose his or her own beliefs onto the patient. The provider should help the patient to explore ideas to provide insight into other options that could be beneficial to that patient. The patient should be praised for all the positive aspects of his or her efforts in taking an active role. Patients need reassurance that they can be successful in meeting their personal goals.

Developing discrepancy can be challenging. Patients need to perceive that there is a difference between where they are and where they want to be. This requires them to have a clear understanding about where they are and to have a set of realistic goals. With the proper approach the provider can help the patient examine and create appropriate goals, without telling the patient what to do or what not to do. This is a trap in to which we can easily fall. This and other traps are further explored later in this text.

Rolling with resistance may be one of the most difficult but most important principles. For many in the healthcare professions it is unnatural to go with a negative flow. From a patient's perspective, to have someone challenge his or her negative thoughts only builds resistance. When the provider allows the patient to explore this resistance, it increases the patient's feelings of acceptance. Feeling acceptance promotes engagement and, ultimately, improves the chances of experiencing a therapeutic encounter.

One useful tool to help better understand motivational interviewing is use of the acronym FRAMES (Britt et al., 2004):

F   Feedback
R   Responsibility is on the patient
A   Advice giving
M   Menu of change options
E   Empathetic style of communication
S   Self-efficacy

Feedback can be provided when the patient elicits it from the provider or when the provider asks permission. The patient must accept responsibility for his or her current situation and choices. Giving advice is an option but may not be welcomed by the patient. When appropriate and accepted, the provider can offer advice. Providing a menu of change options can help to maintain a focus on the task at hand and can decrease stress that occurs when too many options can be overwhelming. Empathy is important to help establish rapport and maintain that rapport between the patient and provider. Self-efficacy is created when the provider empowers the patient and helps the patient to recognize his or her abilities.

As a healthcare provider, it is important to take into consideration what a patient needs. We can only assume what another person needs based on our own experiences. This is not helpful for the patient and can contribute to nonadherence to treatment plans. In a profession such as nursing, there is a misconception that the healthcare provider can and needs to "fix" patients and their problems. This places responsibility on the provider, and we create patients who are either dependent on the provider or are "difficult," meaning one does not listen or follow the recommendations given by the provider. Although frustrating, we unknowingly contribute to this adversarial relationship.

In reality, there is no "difficult patient." Each patient has a history. It is important to explore where they are coming from and who they are to form a relationship. Each person wants to be heard. They want the provider to take an interest in who they are and then walk beside them, coaching and encouraging them to face their personal challenges. How simple it is to recognize that this is an ideal way to interact with our patients, but in actuality there are many barriers that interfere with this type of interaction. These barriers are explored in more detail in Chapter 4.

It is important to recognize that human nature plays a role in each interaction between the nurse and patient. We can expect certain factors to promote or interfere with a **therapeutic relationship**. Both the nurse and patient bring to every encounter preconceptions, past experience, personal beliefs, and expectations. When these factors are congruent, an effective encounter can be anticipated. Often, this is not the case. Although we cannot change some of these factors, we can be aware of them and take them into consideration during each interaction.

Motivational interviewing allows for an interaction to not go smoothly. Whenever the topic of change is on the table, it is natural for there to also be some resistance. Again, human nature plays a role here because change is frightening and it is more comfortable to stay where we are, even if it is not the healthiest option. Change does not always equal comfort, happiness, or even the hope of something positive. So, why change? Change is necessary to prevent many health complications, manage current health issues, or even improve one's present health status. These may be great reasons to change, but the process of change is difficult, to say the least. Resistance does not need to be a negative force. "Resistance is a key to successful treatment if you can recognize it for what it is: an opportunity" (Rollnick, Mason, & Butler, 1999, p. 127). Resistance can be the driving force of the encounter and can give the provider insight into the patient and what is restraining them from change.

Earlier, it was mentioned that we can walk or dance with our patients. Go down their path with them. Do not create the path and expect them to follow. The patient must make some choices independently. Ultimately, it is their life and they know what they need to do. Nurses provide the education to promote healthy lifestyles. What we cannot do is change someone else's behavior. That is a road they have to pave on their own, with guidance and support. Motivational interviewing is a communication, connection, and interaction between nurse and patient. It helps the patient to explore his or her feelings, strengths and weaknesses, and goals. In brief interactions you can do just that.

HOW MOTIVATIONAL INTERVIEWING WORKS

At first glance motivational interviewing is complex. When broken down into simple steps, it appears to be something easily mastered. However, it is indeed complex because people are complex. It is impossible to anticipate what each encounter will bring.

The first step is recognizing that, upon our first encounter, we do not have insight into patients' pasts or thoughts and experiences that shape them and their perspectives. Given this understanding, each time we sit down with a patient we need to take some time to learn more about what they already know, what they would like to or need to know, and the goals they have for that particular encounter. Once that has been established, motivational interviewing guidelines can be used to promote behavior change.

Brief Negotiation Roadmap

Kaiser Permanente has become a leader in the field of training motivational interviewing. Together with Miller and Rollnick, Kaiser Permanente created teaching tools to help the practitioner to participate in brief interventions and effectively promote behavior change. Table 1-1 summarizes the steps involved in motivational interviewing (Roberts, 2005).

Open the Encounter

When first starting a motivational interviewing session, there are some simple yet important factors that should always be included. A brief introduction of who we are and what our role is provides the patient with a background. This is a base on which trust can be built. We need to be clear about what we expect from the encounter and to also clarify what the patient's expectations are. This is important to establish from the start so any misconceptions the nurse or the patient may have can be cleared up before the opportunity to have a positive encounter is negated.

Everyone wants to be heard. Active listening is necessary to provide patients with reassurance that the provider is not only hearing their words but is also listening and processing all that is being said. Body language gives the patient cues that the provider is listening. Reflective listening clarifies that what the provider understands is accurate, allows the patient to clarify any misunderstandings, and

Table 1-1.   Brief Negotiation Roadmap

OPEN THE ENCOUNTER

- Introduce yourself and your role
- Confirm the reason for the visit
- State the appointment length
- Ask Permission

- **Ask** Open-ended question
- **Listen** without judgment or interruption
- **Summarize**/reflect what the patient said
- Information exchange as appropriate

NEGOTIATE THE AGENDA

- **Offer options:** On this chart are a number of things that can affect _____.
- **Elicit patient choice:** Is there one area you would like to focus on today?
  Is there something you'd like to add to the chart, or something else you'd rather talk about?
- Information exchange as appropriate

EXPLORE AMBIVALENCE	ASSESS READINESS
• What are some reasons you would want things to stay the same? *AND* • What are some reasons for making a change? **OR** • What do you like about _____? *AND* • What don't you like about _____? • Summarize	• Ruler or Readiness Scale 0–10 • Straight Question: Why a 5? • Backward Question: Why a 5 and not a 2? • Forward Question: What would need to be different to move you from a 5 to a 7 or 8? • Summarize

TAILOR THE TRANSITION

Not Ready 0–3 • **Raise Awareness** • Elicit Change Talk • Advise & Encourage	• What would need to happen for you to think about changing? • How can I help? • Would you be interested in knowing more about _____? • What might need to be different for you to consider making a change in the future? • Summarize as appropriate
Unsure 4–6 • **Evaluate Ambivalence** • Elicit Change Talk • Build Readiness	• Where does that leave you now? • What do you see as your next steps? • What are you thinking/feeling at this point? • Where does _____ fit into your future? • Summarize as appropriate
Ready 7–10 • **Strengthen Commitment** • Elicit Change Talk • Negotiate a Plan	• What are your main reasons for _____?/Why is this important to you? • What are your ideas for _____? /How might you do it? • How might your life be different when you make this change? • What barriers might you encounter when making this change? • Summarize as appropriate

CLOSE THE ENCOUNTER

- Show appreciation
- Affirm positive behaviors
- Respectfully acknowledge decisions

- **Offer Advice** if appropriate
- **Emphasize Choice**
- **Express Confidence**

- Arrange for follow up and link with available resources

(continues)

Table 1-1. Brief Negotiation Roadmap—continued

INFORMATION EXCHANGE	
Empathic • Supportive of Self-Efficacy • Non-judgmental • Collaborative • Clear and Succinct	
Providing Education • Ask permission • Assess current knowledge • Avoid overwhelming patient with too much information • Check in frequently for understanding • Ask for return demonstration	**Sharing Clinical Results** • Ask permission • Check patient's understanding of the test • Compare results to norms • Ask for patient's interpretation **Sample:** "Your test results are _____. The standard for this test is _____. What do you make of this information?
Offering Advice Give advice only if: • Patient asks • You ask permission • You are professionally bound	**Sample Advice Statement** As a healthcare provider, I strongly encourage you to quit smoking. From my perspective this is the single most important thing you can do for your health. Of course, deciding to quit is your choice. I am confident that should you decide to quit, you will find the method that works best for you.

CONFIDENCE STATEMENT
Genuine • Succinct • Realistic • Supportive of Self-Efficacy
Confidence statements are based on the knowledge that: 1) All people have the capacity to make health behavior change and 2) When they are truly ready to change, they will find a way.
Caution! Avoid the following: • Promoting unachievable or unrealistic expectations • Embedding a judgment, such as confidence that a client will make the 'right' choice • Promoting the clinician's agenda without regard for the client's expressed goals • Offering an expression that is not genuine
Sample Confidence Statements • I am confident that should you decide to begin _____ on a regular basis, you will develop a plan that works for you. • I feel certain that if you choose to _____ you will find a way to make it happen. • From our conversation today, it is clear to me that if you decide to _____ you will be able to create an approach that is effective for you. • I am confident that your _____ (enthusiasm, determination, success with other lifestyle changes....) will be of great value as you begin to work on this plan. • I feel very positive that if you choose to _____, you will formulate a strategy that is practical for you.

© 2005. The Permanente Medical Group, Inc., Kaiser Permanente. Created by Sandra Roberts, RN. All Rights Reserved. Used With Permission.

gives the patient reassurance that he or she is understood (Rollnick, Miller, & Butler, 2008). Summarizing what the patient has said increases the patient's confidence in the provider because he or she knows that what was said is validated.

The importance of listening should not dissuade the practitioner from participating in the conversation. If the patient asks questions, answers should be objective and not impart the practitioner's beliefs onto the patient. If there is information that may be important for patients to know so they can make informed decisions, it is important to ask the patient if it is okay to share some information. Simply asking permission keeps the encounter client focused and demonstrates a lack of assumption that the patient wants input from the practitioner.

After permission is granted by the patient, the communication needs to remain open. Asking close-ended questions can end a conversation abruptly. Open-ended questions allow the patient to expand upon his or her thoughts. Patients should do the majority of the talking, but some open-ended questions are useful in bringing more from patients to further explore who they are, what they know, what they believe they need to know, and what their goals are. It can be an invitation to a relationship between the patient and the provider (Rollnick et al., 2008).

Negotiate the Agenda

There needs to be patient participation in determining the path of the encounter. Negotiating is like dancing with the patient, and when both the patient and provider are taking the same steps, they can create a masterpiece (Rollnick et al., 1999). Asking what they would like to focus on encourages patients to work on what is important to them. If an encounter is based on what the provider believes is important and is not related to the patient's agenda, the encounter will not be successful. The patient may have a number of issues on which he or she would like to focus. The provider should offer options so the patient can choose and remain self-efficacious. Sharing information, with permission, may be helpful for the patient to decide the focus of the encounter.

Assess Readiness

Not every patient that comes to an encounter is ready to make behavioral changes. The readiness scale of 0 to 10 is a tool that can assess how ready the patient is at the time of the encounter. For example, the patient may decide to have weight loss on the agenda. The provider can ask, "On a scale of 0 to 10, how ready are you to work on losing weight?" The patient responds with a level of 6. The provider could ask why that patient believes he or she is at that particular place. Another approach is to ask why the patient did not choose a lower number. This puts a focus on some of the positive reasons the patient may believe he or she is at during the time of the encounter. Exploring why they are not at a higher level allows patients to explore some of the things standing in their way to initiate change. Again, summarizing what they say verifies the provider's comprehension of the patient's level of motivation.

Explore Ambivalence

People often get stuck in the realm of ambivalence. We know what we need to do and we want to do it, but we have a list of things getting in the way of making a change. "I can't exercise because I don't have the time." Exploring those barriers to why there is no time or why the behavior change is not possible can promote thoughts on how to overcome those hurdles. Continuing with open-ended questions, the provider can inquire about what would be beneficial for making a behavior change. This shifts the focus from what is standing in the way to why the change is important. Again, summary of the information exchanged promotes a positive encounter.

Tailor the Transition

After exploring ambivalence and assessing readiness to change, the provider can tailor the transition with the hope to elicit **change talk**. When the patient is at levels 0–3 on the readiness scale, he or she is clearly not ready to make a behavioral change. The role of the provider at this time is to raise awareness about the issue so an informed choice can be made. Sharing information, with permission, can be useful here. Table 1-1 provides examples of questions that can be asked that help elicit change talk and moving farther along the readiness scale (Roberts, 2005). Encouraging the patient and offering support prove effective in validating their current status, if nothing else.

Level 4–6 on the readiness scale is the stage of ambivalence. Patients are not sure they are ready to make solid steps toward change. With some guided interaction patients can raise their level of readiness. Examples of questions to elicit change talk are available in Table 1-1 (Roberts, 2005). This is a most challenging stage because patients often feel stuck. They are not confident in their ability to change, may lack information about how to change or what needs to change, or may just lack the resources necessary to make a behavioral change. Further exploration of this ambivalence can raise the level of readiness.

When patients come to you at level 7–10 on the readiness scale, they are ready and motivated to make a behavioral change. Eliciting change talk is easier, and you can build on the patient's current momentum. The goal here is to have the patient commit to some actions to reach his or her goal. Table 1-1 provides examples of open-ended questions that can gain that commitment (Roberts, 2005). Negotiation is necessary for the encounter to remain client centered when creating a plan for the patient to follow. The plan should be based on what the patient believes will work in his or her current lifestyle or situation.

Throughout this phase the patient and provider can explore the "if," "but," and "why/why not." Helping to find what is holding the patient back can open doors for what could help him or her move forward. Summarizing what the patient says is important to validate that the provider is listening and understanding the patient perspective.

Close the Encounter

Closing an encounter comes with its own challenges. Knowing when the attempts to elicit change talk have been exhausted or a commitment has been made is important. Summarizing all that has occurred in the encounter can offer one last chance to clear up any misconceptions and build the relationship between the patient and provider. Saying a simple "thank you" for sharing their perspectives or sharing a piece of their personal experience can express appreciation and respect for the patient as a person and for his or her decisions. Giving praise provides affirmation that a patient's feelings and thoughts have not been criticized and maintains a nonjudgmental environment.

When ending the encounter it is okay to offer advice. By this time a relationship has been established and permission has been granted. Reinforce that the patient has choices. Telling the patient you are confident in his or her success in making the behavior change adds to the momentum and increases confidence. Making plans for the next encounter can be negotiated at this time.

Information Exchange

Motivational interviewing takes on the flow of a natural conversation. There are a few key aspects to exchanging information. This can be in the form of educating, sharing clinical-related information, and providing advice. Information can be elicited by patients when they feel there is information they need or the provider may find information would be useful after assessing patients' current level of understanding. Permission should always be requested when offering to share information with the patient. Reassessing for understanding can help clarify any misconceptions or need for further information sharing.

Often, the patient has had a clinical evaluation and may need to know results of a test or findings from a physical exam. With permission, these findings can be shared with the patient. The provider cannot assume that the patient understands what tests were done or what is normal or abnormal. This is another opportunity to assess level of understanding to help determine what information needs to be further explained. Reassessing what these findings mean to the patient can assist in exploring how this information fits into the patient's present goals or lack of goals.

Opportunities arise where the provider has some advice he or she believes may be helpful or even necessary to share with a patient. As with any information the provider has to offer, permission should be sought. If the patient asks the provider for advice, that permission is assumed. See Table 1-1 for a sample advice statement (Roberts, 2005).

Confidence Statement

Sharing provider confidence in the patient reinforces a current confidence level or potentially creates a level of confidence that is not currently there. You may find that an encounter flowed with resistance and the patient remains non-committal. It is important to find something positive from the interaction, such as "you have really worked hard to understand your condition, but still feel a lack of control. I am confident that when you find that piece that you have in your power to work on, you will be successful." Other examples of confidence statements can be found in Table 1-1 (Roberts, 2005).

SUMMARY

Miller and Rollnick created an effective tool in motivational interviewing. A brief explanation has been provided here and is only a stepping stone to promoting behavior change in our patients. Therapeutic communication is important in each and every interaction. Time is often short when the patient and provider meet. Although complex, the basic principles can guide us, and mastery can be obtained. Although this tactic was only created as recently as 1983, it is a growing concept and can be used across different healthcare practices. Motivational interviewing is a form of communication that allows patient involvement, respect for each patient as an individual with his or her own agenda, and acceptance of the patient's choices. This is the dance. Let the patient choose the music, dance, or choose to sit out and be thankful for the opportunity to participate in that patient's personal journey toward behavior change.

REFERENCES

Britt, E., Hudson, S. M., & Blampied, N. M. (2004). Motivational interviewing in health settings: A review. *Patient Education and Counseling, 53,* 147–155.

Kumm, S., Hicks, V., Shupe, S., & Hagemaster, J. (2002). You can help your clients change. *Dimensions of Critical Care Nursing, 21*(2), 72–77.

Lange, N., & Tigges, B. B. (2005). Influence positive change with motivational interviewing. *The Nurse Practitioner, 30*(3), 44–53.

Levensky, E. R., Forcehimes, A., O'Donohue, W. T., & Beitz, K. (2007). Motivational interviewing: An evidence-based approach to counseling helps patients follow treatment recommendations. *American Journal of Nursing, 107*(10), 50–58.

Miller, W. R. (1996). Motivational interviewing: Research, practice and puzzles. *Addictive Behaviors, 21*(6), 835–842.

Miller, W. R., & Rollnick, S. (2002). *Motivational interviewing: Preparing people for change.* New York: The Guilford Press.

Miller, W.R., Zweben, A., DiClemente, C.C., & Rychtarik, R.G. (1992). *Motivational enhancement therapy manual: A clinical research guide for therapists treating individuals with alcohol abuse and dependence.* Rockville, MD: National Institute on Alcohol Abuse and Alcoholism.

Rolfe, G. (2004). Motivational interviewing: A hammer looking for a nail? *Journal of Psychiatric and Mental Health Nursing, 11,* 494–501.

Roberts, S. (2005). *Communication for health action: Motivating change* (3rd ed.). The Permanente Medical Group.

Rollnick, S., Mason, P., & Butler, C. (1999). *Health behavior change: A guide for practitioners.* Edinburgh: Churchill Livingstone.

Rollnick, S., & Miller, W. R. (1995). What is motivational interviewing? *Behavioural and Cognitive Psychotherapy, 23,* 325–334.

Rollnick, S., Miller, W. R., & Butler, C. C. (2008). *Motivational interviewing in health care: Helping patients change behavior.* New York: The Guilford Press.

Shinitzky, H. E., & Kub, J. (2001). The art of motivating behavior change: The use of motivational interviewing to promote health. *Public Health Nursing, 18*(3), 178–185.

CHAPTER 2

Making the Pieces Fit: Therapeutic Communication and the Nursing Process

---

OBJECTIVES

After completing this chapter, the reader will be able to

1. Identify five forms of therapeutic communication.
2. Ask an open-ended question.
3. Create a reflective statement.
4. Explain how therapeutic communication plays a role in motivational interviewing.
5. Provide examples of how motivational interviewing fits into each step of the nursing process.

KEY TERMS

Change talk
Nursing process
OARS

Therapeutic communication
Therapeutic relationship

ROLE OF THERAPEUTIC COMMUNICATION IN MOTIVATIONAL INTERVIEWING

Therapeutic communication has always played a vital role in nursing practice. It is a respectful way of communicating. It is a way to show we are listening. It is a way to show we care. It is an expression of empathy. Although it is at the very root of nursing, it can be overshadowed by what may appear to be more important. Studies have been done on communication, and although some were based on the premise that compliance is related to information provided by the nurse, the result is most successful when nurses and patients negotiate and agree on treatment goals (Rollnick, Mason, & Butler, 1999). With all the restrictions,

15

high expectations, and long hours nurses put into their careers, it is no wonder effective communication is often lacking. In the rush of the workday, there is little time to chat with our patients. A **therapeutic relationship**, one in which the patient feels comfortable being open and honest with the nurse, depends on therapeutic communication. A therapeutic relationship is one in which trust, co-existence, self-awareness, and empathy exist (Welch, 2005). In reality, what is often communicated by the nurse tends to be brief and hurried. Intermittent reminders of how to communicate effectively can help enhance our communication skills. This section reviews the key aspects of therapeutic communication.

"Communication is both verbal and nonverbal and occurs within an environmental context of cultural, family, and individual life experiences" (Haber, McMahon, Price-Hoskins, & Sileau, 1992, p. 132). Who we are and our past experiences all affect how we communicate, both verbally and nonverbally. Verbal and nonverbal communication skills are often overlooked because they require self-awareness. We know about these skills, we are aware of how others use these skills, but we do not always see how well we practice what we know. Personality, temperament, and communication skills of those we are talking with can significantly affect how we communicate. To enhance our own communication skills, we can review what the skills are and practice them. To increase self-awareness, we can role play or work with someone who can offer open and honest criticism.

The acronym is helpful in breaking down the communication into manageable pieces (Miller & Rollnick, 2002):

O Open-ended questions
A Affirmation
R Reflection
S Summary

Table 2-1 provides some examples of OARS. Here we review these and some nonverbal skills to improve effective communication between the nurse and patient.

Verbal Communication

Verbal communication is more than just the words we speak. Choice of words is important, but there are some other aspects that are just as pertinent, if not more so. Tone of voice can impact the direction a conversation will go. Consider the following statement: "I'd like to hear how you are doing today." The words are clearly opening up the conversation with an interest in how the patient is doing. Imagine the tone of voice. It can be friendly and inviting by using a quiet relaxed tone. It can also be uninviting when the tone is heavy and monotone, which actually demonstrates a disinterest on the part of the nurse. When we are hurried, we can become unaware of the tone of voice we use. The tone of voice sets the climate of the entire conversation and reveals the speaker's attitude and assumptions about the current topic (Rollnick, Miller, & Butler, 2008).

Table 2-1.　Examples of OARS

Open-Ended Questions	Affirmation	Reflection	Summary
Could you share with me what has worked for you in the past when faced with a similar situation?	You have worked very hard to get to this point.	Previously, you said you wanted to . . . , but truly you are afraid of making the changes to reach that goal.	Throughout our conversation you have said you would like to . . . . . and will accomplish this by . . . . . in this amount of time.
What are your current plans to accomplish your goal?	You should be commended for all your positive efforts in meeting your goals.	On one hand you are happy with your current lifestyle, but on the other hand you realize that some changes need to be made.	I would like to review what we talked about today.
What do you believe you can accomplish at this time?	It is obvious you have invested a lot into making these changes.	You have worked on . . . . . in the past and been unsuccessful and now you are afraid to try again because you could fail.	To summarize what you just said . . . . .
How do you believe it will feel to accomplish your goal?	You have faced many challenges along the way, but you did not give up and now you are reaping the rewards.	Making a change is never easy and you realize that you will have to put forth quite a bit of effort to accomplish your goals.	We covered a lot today and I would like to review what we discussed.

The questions we ask also need to be considered. Questions should be limited so that listening can occur and so the nurse does not direct where the interaction goes (Rollnick et al., 2008). When a question requires only a yes or no answer, this often leads to a one-sided conversation. The person asking these close-ended questions dominates the conversation and does not meet the goal of therapeutic communication. Open-ended questions require the person to thoughtfully consider the answer and opens it up so the nurse and patient can have communication back and forth. We could ask a patient if they have any pain and they will likely answer yes or no, but that does not give us any insight to the level or intensity of the pain. A better way to ask about pain might be, "Could you tell me about your pain?" The patient is likely to respond with more details about their pain. The conversation may go like this:

Patient: "I didn't have any pain last night, but this morning the pain is unbearable."

Nurse: "How would you describe your pain?"

Patient: "The pain is sharp and goes from my back down the leg to my toes."

When questions are asked in a way that encourages the patient to provide more information, the patient will share more information they find to be relevant and the conversation does not have to be one of the nurse going through a list of questions with the patient answering yes or no each time. The information the nurse gains can be invaluable. "Questions should be designed to help the client clarify his own problems, rather than provide information to the interviewer" (Bolton, 1979, p. 45).

When attempting to maintain a patient-centered focus, we may need to ask for clarification. Not only will this help the nurse to better understand what the patient is saying, it reinforces for the patient that the nurse is listening and interested in what they are saying (Stone, Patton, & Heen, 1999). One way to clarify the information is to use reflection statements. The patient may share a lot of information in a short period of time. It is important to sift through the information and get to the heart of the conversation and use that information when reflecting back to the patient. Consider the following conversation:

Nurse: "I see that you are here today to talk with me about stress management."

Patient: "Yes, I have been struggling with a lot of anxiety and it is hard for me to stay focused on anything. I just get so overwhelmed with everything going on in my life that I can't get anything accomplished. I got up this morning and had a ton of things to do, but just sat there for about an hour because I couldn't think of what I needed to do or where to even start."

Nurse: "You have so much going on that it is hard to keep organized and that is causing you to feel anxious."

Patient: "That is exactly what I mean. And I have tried keeping lists and making schedules, but nothing is working."

In that conversation the nurse was able to clarify what the patient was saying and to help her focus on the problem at hand. One skill the nurse must have is to find the focus and identify what the root of the problem may be. The key here is to listen to what the patient identifies as the problem and not to impose our beliefs when identifying the problem. There may be times when a patient has multiple concerns and may benefit from help focusing on one issue at a time. In the previous conversation the patient knew she was anxious and overwhelmed, so the problem is easily identified. The next conversation may be more difficult to sort out and identify the problem.

Nurse: "Good morning. I see you are here because you are having some difficulty sleeping. Maybe you could tell me a little more about that."

Patient: "Well, I just haven't been sleeping well for the past 3 weeks."

Nurse: "What are your thoughts on what is going on?"

Patient: "I don't know. I try to go to sleep and I just lay there for hours and can't stop thinking of everything I need to get done during the day, and then I'll sleep for a couple hours and wake up with my mind spinning about all I am responsible for."

Nurse: "So, you have a hard time quieting your thoughts enough to get a good night of rest."

Patient: "Yes, that is true."

Nurse: "You have a lot on your plate and it is hard to break it down to manageable pieces."

Patient: "I do. I have just started a new job, I have my family I am responsible for, there is always a crisis to deal with, and there is never a moment for me to just relax. I just can't relax."

Nurse: "So, let me clarify what you are saying. You have a lot of responsibilities and they are overwhelming. It is hard to prioritize and find a balance, so it is now interfering with your sleep."

Patient: "That is exactly what I am saying."

In this conversation the nurse not only clarified what the patient is saying but helped the patient to focus on the problem at hand. Sometimes the problem is not clear to the patient but is more easily identified by the nurse, just by listening. The important thing is not to tell the patient what the problem is but to help them identify the problem. In keeping with a patient focus, the agenda should be set by the patient based on his or her interpretation of the problem. The patient may come to you with something he or she identified as a problem, but without clarification and further exploration it may not be well communicated to the nurse and the nurse may inaccurately assess what the true problem is (Rollnick et al., 2008).

There may be times when a problem is not the reason for the conversation. The patient may need reinforcement or affirmation that what they are doing is the right thing. Positive reinforcement enhances the patient's momentum to keep on the right track. There is always room to improve where we are, but we need to accept when people are happy with where they are in the current moment. They may have found a way to make things work for them and not be interested in further changes. Offering praise and using positive statements is essential to building self-efficacy and promote motivation. "Self efficacy refers to a person's confidence in his or her ability to make a specific change in behavior" (Rollnick et al., 1999, p. 92). Imagine you worked very hard at losing weight and someone tells you that you can do better or you did not lose enough weight. It is detrimental to our self-perception and sheds a negative light on all the hard work we have put into meeting our personal goals. It is more important to light the path than to blow out the candles.

As nurses, we are always looking for that "teachable moment" when the patient is receptive to learning and the nurse can jump in and offer information to improve his or her health or overall well-being (Bastable, 2006). Information sharing is acceptable if the patient wants the information. So often we give information to patients because we believe they need the information to promote a healthier lifestyle. If the information is not sought out, the information is often not retained and, in fact, often leads to resistance (Rollnick et al., 2008). Always seek permission from the patient before offering unsolicited information. Consider a patient who has just had a heart attack, is obese, and has hypertension, dyslipidemia, and type 2 diabetes. There are many teachable topics for this person. Here is a possible conversation between the nurse and patient:

> Nurse: "Good morning. I am here to help you with your discharge planning. What concerns do you have that we can address before you are discharged?"
>
> Patient: "Well, I'd like to be discharged right away. My husband is not well and I need to get home to attend to him."
>
> Nurse: "It must be very difficult to focus on your own health when you are worried about your husband."
>
> Patient: "That's for sure. I don't have time to worry about me. I just know I need to get home as soon as possible."
>
> Nurse: "Share with me a little about what is involved in the care for your husband, and together maybe we could come up with some ways to help you both."
>
> Patient: "Well, I have to make all his meals and feed him if he is having a bad day and can't or won't feed himself. I have to make sure he gets his medicine and shower, and if I'm lucky, I might be able to get him out of the house for a little fresh air. The doctor told me I am doing all the things for my husband that I should be doing for me so I don't have another heart attack. I just can't take care of myself and him at the same time."
>
> Nurse: "Would you like me to share with you how some other people have found ways to manage situations like yours?"
>
> Patient: "Sure. I would love to hear any suggestions you may have."

Asking permission allowed the patient to determine if the information was something she wanted. The nurse asked in a respectful way and allowed the choice to be made by the patient, keeping the conversation patient centered. The conversation could have ended more abruptly if the nurse came in and told the patient "this is what you need to do" because the patient is more concerned about her husband.

Humor, when appropriate and respectful, can be used in therapeutic communication. Keep in mind that people often use humor when they are nervous or concerned about something. Humor helps to relieve anxiety but also may be used for avoidance of true feelings. Take the time to try to determine if the use of humor is part of a patient's normal temperament or a defense mechanism. Knowing this can determine if the conversation succeeds or fails.

Patients often ask advice from nurses. Advice sharing should be limited. Our perceptions come from our own belief system and may not fit with the patient's beliefs. Remember to keep the conversations nonjudgmental, which is difficult if the nurse shares personal views. "We often seek to get feelings out of the way by 'fixing' them" (Stone et al., 1999, p. 106). It is one matter to acknowledge the patient's feelings and another to inflict our feelings onto the patient. Expressing personal feelings, judgment, giving advice, or providing solutions interfere with effective listening and, ultimately, with therapeutic communication (Roberts, 2005). Nurses need to be a resource for patients, without inflicting their own personal views or opinions onto the patient.

Nonverbal Communication

Whereas verbal communication is there to be heard, processed in our minds, and verbally responded to, nonverbal communication is not so obvious. It can be difficult to "read" nonverbal cues. Researchers found that 75% of what is heard is not fully understood, is forgotten, or is simply ignored. This clarifies our general lack of ability to fully attend to the spoken word (Bolton, 1979). Just as important as verbal communication, nonverbal communication has a direct impact on how a conversation proceeds. Nonverbal communication can contribute to the meaning behind the spoken words or send a message alone (Haber et al., 1992). The most important form of nonverbal communication is listening. Listening is not only processing what is being said, it is also being aware of the other person's nonverbal cues. What they are saying may have a whole different meaning when you take into consideration what they are not saying. The key is to listen with both your ears and your eyes. Listen actively.

Active listening encompasses a whole range of facial expressions and body language. Being self-aware of expressions and body language helps promote a therapeutic interaction. To become more self-aware we can use a mirror, video tape ourselves in conversation, and role play with others who will offer honest criticism to help enhance our skills. Nodding your head, use of facial expressions at appropriate times, and good eye contact can be used to demonstrate active listening. Body positioning is also key to showing the patient you are listening and being nonjudgmental. Crossing of arms and constant movement of hands and legs will be interpreted as lack of interest or of concentration. The key is self-awareness.

Silence is a nonverbal tool that is difficult to use. Often, we believe silence needs to be masked by chatter. The question is what happens during that silence. For the person listening, it is often difficult to remain silent and not keep the conversation going. We often believe we need to fill the gaps in the conversation. It can feel uncomfortable to remain silent. Time is valuable and we feel it is wasted on silence. What is important to understand about silence is that it is a positive tool. It allows the person talking to take a moment to recollect his or her thoughts or consider his or her next statement. When we fill that gap with chatter, we take away that opportunity for thought. When we allow the silence, we are letting the person know we are patiently waiting for what he or she has to say next. As uncomfortable as it may be, it is important to practice this skill, because it allows the person talking to take that moment to decide if there is more to share. Silence tells the patient you are interested in hearing more (Bolton, 1979).

It is essential to be aware of how we communicate both verbally and nonverbally, to communicate therapeutically with others. Verbal and nonverbal communication must always be congruent. When verbal and nonverbal cues are succinct, they validate one another, but if they contradict one another there is confusion (Haber et al., 1992) (Figure 2-1). Validation keeps the conversation

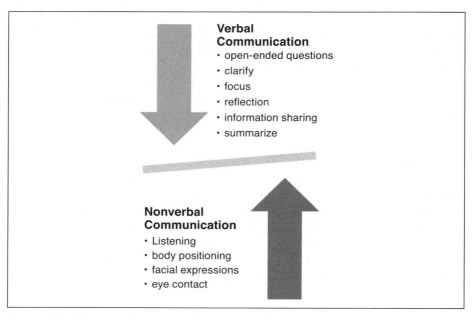

Figure 2-1   Therapeutic Communication

going, whereas contradiction shuts down communication. Once it is lost, it is difficult to recover the trust and respect to develop a therapeutic relationship.

INCORPORATION OF MOTIVATIONAL INTERVIEWING INTO NURSING PRACTICE

Motivational interviewing fits perfectly into the nursing profession. As coaches, therapists, care providers, and educators we need a caring, respectful tool to promote behavior change, and motivational interviewing is such a tool. By looking at each step of the nursing process we can see how it fits. Many areas of nursing have already proven its effectiveness. Many other areas of nursing can and will benefit from the use of motivational interviewing.

Motivational Interviewing and the Nursing Process

The compass that guides nurses in their practice is the nursing process. To determine if motivational interviewing fits into the nursing spectrum, we must look at each step of the nursing process (Figure 2-2). "The nursing process is a thoughtful, deliberate use of a problem-solving approach to nursing" (Ellis, Nowlis, & Bentz, 1992, p. 9).

Assessment

The first step in the nursing process is to assess or investigate. This occurs in motivational interviewing when the conversation begins right through to the end of the encounter. The nurse must always be attentive to where the patient is mentally and physically. "Assessment of the individual client in the context of health promotion expands beyond physical assessment to also include a comprehensive examination of other client health parameters, health beliefs, and health behaviors" (Pender, Murdaugh, & Parsons, 2002, p. 119). We use all of our senses to assess a patient. Clinically, we look for symmetry, auscultate for clear succinct sounds, palpate for lumps or masses, and percuss for tympany. In communication we look, listen, and feel for the patient to take interest in their health care, for that moment of clarity where the nurse and patient are in the same place. This is when the nurse is cheerleading and the patient is running with the ball. The patient is looking to make a change in behavior or to take steps toward a healthier lifestyle and the nurse is assessing the patient's readiness to change.

The nurse assesses a number of things throughout a conversation. The nurse should be looking to answer the following questions:

- What does this patient need right now? (This is what the patient believes he or she needs at this moment.)

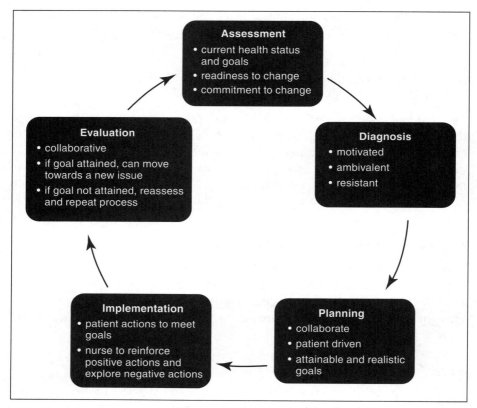

Figure 2-2 The Nursing Process and Motivational Interviewing

- Is the patient engaged in this conversation?
- What do the patient's verbal and nonverbal cues tell the nurse?
- Is the present concern a stepping stone to a larger goal?
- What is getting in the way for this patient to achieve the goal?
- Is the patient ready to change? And if not, where is he or she on the readiness to change continuum?
- What are they willing to change to attain their goal?
- How committed/motivated are they to change?
- What does the patient need from the nurse at this time? (This could be reassurance, education, resources, or counseling, etc.)
- Am I promoting therapeutic communication through verbal and nonverbal cues?
- Am I remaining nonjudgmental and keeping my personal views out of the conversation?

During the assessment the nurse's task is to elicit information. This can be accomplished by asking questions, reflecting, and listening. The nurse must find out what the patient's concerns are and determine what contributes to the problem, what may help the problem, and how it may be resolved. With motivational interviewing the nurse encourages the patient to participate, if not take responsibility, in his or her health care. Questions asked by the nurse should be limited to promote therapeutic communication within the motivational interviewing model. The following are examples of an assessment with and without the tools of motivational interviewing:

Example 1:

Nurse: "Good morning. I understand you are here today to talk about smoking cessation."

Patient: "Yes. My doctor says I need to quit and I know I should, but it is too hard."

Nurse: "Well, your doctor knows how important it is to your health to stop smoking."

Patient: "I just don't think I can do it."

Nurse: "I'm going to give you some information and we will talk about everything you need to do to stop smoking."

Example 2:

Nurse: "Good morning. I understand you are here today to talk about smoking cessation."

Patient: "Yes. My doctor says I need to quit and I know I should, but it is too hard."

Nurse: "What do you think makes it so difficult for you?"

Patient: "I've been smoking for 40 years and it's hard to change something you've done for so long."

Nurse: Silence

Patient: "See, I've tried to quit before and I always went back to it. Something would happen to stress me out and I guess that is one way I cope with stress. I have a cigarette."

Nurse: "On one hand you want to quit smoking, but on the other hand you have done it for so long and been unsuccessful when you tried to quit in the past that you feel it may be too difficult to quit."

Patient: "That's exactly it, but stress gets to me every time."

Nurse: "You are saying that smoking is a way of dealing with stress. I'm curious if you can remember any time that you have used another tool to cope with stress."

Patient: "Oh yeah. I used to go for a walk when I got stressed. And I'd have a cigarette as soon as I got home."

Nurse: "Walking helped but did not fully relieve the stress."

Patient: "No. But maybe I could try walking when I feel like I need a cigarette. I just don't know what I would do when I got home and wanted a cigarette."

Nurse: "You are trying to find another distraction when you get home from your walk. Would you like me to share with you some tools other people have used to distract themselves to avoid smoking?"

In the first example the conversation is brief and the only assessment is in clarifying the problem. In the second example the nurse assesses the patient throughout the conversation by using reflective statements, silence, or simply restating what the patient is saying. The nurse ascertains what the patient is there for, the patient's goal and the barriers to reaching that goal and inquires if the patient is interested in getting some information to help attain their goal.

Diagnosis

To diagnose is to identify the problem. Clinically, this may be simple, such as increased weight gain or decreased mobility. In motivational interviewing the diagnosis may be a little more difficult. In conversation, the topic may initially appear to be about one thing, yet as you continue the patient may identify a completely different problem that takes priority. The key is to pay attention to the patient and what he or she is saying verbally and nonverbally. For example, a patient may be looking for information about weight loss, but through careful assessment the nurse may find that a foot ulcer is the primary concern and needs to be addressed before working toward weight loss. It is important not to create our own agenda. If we walk with the patient and let them guide the encounter, the answers to our questions will be answered.

Motivational interviewing is the key that opens the door for behavior change. Through assessment, the nurse can determine a diagnosis of motivation, ambivalence, or resistance to change. The diagnosis of motivation is the least challenging because when someone is motivated, it is a much quicker path through the remaining steps of the nursing process. They may have already thought of how they may proceed with changing a particular behavior. Often, a patient is ambivalent about making changes or even seeing a need to make a change. Behind motivational interviewing is the belief that most people are unsure about making a change and the focus should be on resolving that ambivalence (Miller & Rollnick, 2003). When this is the case, the nurse explores the source of the ambivalence. It is helpful to encourage the patient to explore the positive and negative aspects of the present behavior and the possibility of changing that behavior. The ideal result is for the patient to move closer to motivation and, ultimately, a commitment to change. Many patients are resistant to change. Change is difficult and can be frightening because change brings forth the unknown. Resistance can simply be due to a lack of information or can be as complicated as a person's negative past experience. Each person falls somewhere along the continuum between resistance, ambivalence, and motivation.

Motivation is what drives us to make choices and take actions. The reasons for motivation are endless, but these reasons can offer insight into what direction the patient will go and how successful he or she may be in changing behavior. Motivation can be broken down into intrinsic versus extrinsic. Our internal motivators can range from wanting to improve health, to wanting to gain more knowledge, to wanting to avoid complications of a present illness. External motivators may come from watching a loved one suffer and hoping to avoid a similar experience or from a loved one's urging for the patient to change. "Motivation is not regarded as an individual trait that is difficult to change but as a state that is changeable and influenced by the practitioner's interviewing style" (Botelho, 2004, p. 103).

Ambivalence is feeling two ways about something (Miller & Rollnick, 2002). For example, a person knows he or she needs to take medicine but at the same time is worried about side effects. The word "but" is often a trigger to identify when someone is ambivalent. The problem with ambivalence is that we often get "stuck" there and are unable to move in any direction. The nurse's role here is to help the patient get past this stage and into **change talk**. Change talk is when the patient verbalizes that he or she is considering making positive steps toward behavior change (Rollnick et al., 2008). A variety of ways for the nurse to elicit change talk when a patient is ambivalent follows (Roberts, 2005; Miller & Rollnick, 2002):

- Explore the positives and negatives of not making a change
- Explore the positives and negatives of making a change
- Allow time for the patient to explore their feelings
- Be patient because ambivalence can be difficult to resolve.

Resistance is a common phenomenon when dealing with behavior change. Resistance varies by degree and timing for each individual (Schenk & Hartley, 2002). Without realizing it the nurse may be confrontational, and a cycle begins. The patient resists and the nurse confronts even more, causing the patient to resist even stronger. Maintaining empathy, understanding, and a nonjudgmental attitude is best when faced with resistance. When recognized, it should be explored for an understanding of why the patient is resisting. Once that is established, the resistance will decrease and the possibility for change will increase (Botelho, 2004). In Chapter 4, more tools to deal with resistance are explored.

Planning

Nurses are accustomed to identifying steps the nurse and patient should take to improve the problem that was diagnosed. In motivational interviewing the patient participates in the planning. Often, patients do most of the planning themselves with little input from the nurse. This can be difficult to let go of the control we once had in the planning process. Consider having someone tell you what you need to do to fix a problem and it is not a realistic solution for you and your lifestyle or beliefs. Likely nothing will change because it is more difficult to try something and fail than to not try at all. Now consider having the ability to help plan the changes. You know a few steps you can take that you can follow through with. You are more likely to take those steps than take steps that you believe are not within your grasp.

During the planning phase of the **nursing process** it is vital to create a plan together. This plan should provide direction to meet the patient's goals but should not dictate what the nurse believes the goals should be. The goals should be attainable and realistic based on the patient's knowledge, abilities, and motives. As a team the nurse and patient devise this plan that will be the basis from which the patient works from toward meeting his or her goals (Pender et al., 2002).

The following is an example of a nurse–patient encounter that exemplifies the planning stage of the nursing process through motivational interviewing:

> Nurse: "To summarize what you have said, you would like to increase the amount of exercise you do to help you achieve a 5- to 7-pound weight loss each month until you achieve a total 30-pound weight loss."
>
> Patient: "Yes. I would like to begin an exercise program, but I'm not sure where to begin."
>
> Nurse: "Starting out is always challenging."
>
> Patient: "It is. I would really like to walk more but have heard that working out with weights would be really good, too."
>
> Nurse: "I would love to hear what ideas you have for an exercise schedule."
>
> Patient: "I was thinking that I could either walk at least 4 days a week for a half hour each time. But I also thought I could try to walk 2 or 3 days and spend another 2 or 3 days with weight training, if I could go to the gym a few times a week."
>
> Nurse: "It is often difficult to get out and go to a gym routinely."
>
> Patient: "Well, kind of. I used to do it but got out of the routine. I should be able to do it again. That is what I will do. I will walk and do some weight training and balance it out so I get a total of 5 or 6 days a week."

By using the tools of motivational interviewing, the nurse was able to elicit from the patient a detailed goal of how he was going to address his problem of being overweight.

Implementation

The implementation stage is a time to follow through with the actions required to meet the patient's goals. Originally, nurses used the implementation phase to carry out the treatment goals the nurse created to meet the patient's needs (Ellis et al., 1992). In motivational interviewing it is the patient who is taking action in the implementation phase. When the patient starts implementing these goals, the nurse's role is to reinforce the positive efforts and explore the negative aspects. The actions required to attain the goals are primarily for the patient to accomplish. This is where behavior change begins for the patient. During this step the nurse may provide education to help attain a goal. If the patient falters in his or her commitment, the nurse will strive to strengthen that commitment and keep the momentum going. The patient will go through transitions and will need the nurse to continue assessing and reassessing, possibly going through the nursing process repeatedly to address one issue.

The nurse's role depends on how the patient is progressing. An encounter during this stage could reveal problems the patient has found in his initial goal. In the previous nurse–patient conversation the patient created a goal of working out 5 to 6 days a week. During the next conversation, however, the patient may be struggling to implement the goal as it was stated.

> Nurse: "We are here today to follow up and see how you are doing with your exercise routine."
> Patient: "I have been trying. I get out and walk at least 2 days a week, but most of the time I walk three times a week. I have had a hard time doing the weight training because I can't afford the costs of the gym."
> Nurse: "That is great that you are walking. I'm sorry to hear that you are having a difficult time being able to find an affordable place to work out."
> Patient: "I checked out the local gyms and they all want so much money, and I just don't have that kind of money to spend."
> Nurse: "Would you like me to share with you some ways to decrease the costs or find places that are more affordable?"
> Patient: "I would really appreciate that."

In this encounter the nurse not only praised the positive efforts and elicited additional information about the barriers, but also asked permission to share some ideas to overcome the barriers. The nurse assessed what the problem was for the patient to complete the implementation stage and was then able to help the patient find solutions to proceed with implementing his personal goal.

Evaluation

Evaluation is the process of reassessing and determining if the goal was accomplished, a new goal needs to be made to address the original problem, or if there is a different problem that takes precedence. Together, the nurse and patient determine if goals were attained (Pender et al., 2002). This stage allows evaluation of what has been effective and what has not. The importance of this stage lies in which direction the encounter goes. This could be the end of the original problem and assessment of a separate problem. If the original problem has not been resolved, the communication will focus on reassessing the original problem and creating either a new diagnosis or a new plan of action. The following interaction demonstrates some possibilities:

> Nurse: "Well, it has been 3 months since you began working toward your goal of weight loss. How would you say things have been going?"
> Patient: "I have been able to lose 5 pounds a month, which was what I set out to do."
> Nurse: "Congratulations. You have worked very hard to achieve your goal and you can see the positive effects of your efforts."
> Patient: "Thank you. It wasn't easy, but I'm glad I did it and will now be able to keep going with it. I just think I would do better with it, if I could only work on the nutrition side of things."
> Nurse: "Nutrition proves to be challenging for many people. Would you mind sharing with me what you find most difficult in managing your nutrition?"
> Patient: "I just can't seem to give up the sweets."

In this interaction the patient has accomplished the goal but wants to create another goal to improve his nutrition to enhance his success with resolving the original problem. Consider a different scenario:

> Nurse: "Well, it has been 3 months since you began working toward your goal of weight loss. How would you say things are going?"
> Patient: "Not so good. The first month I lost 8 pounds, but the last 2 months I have only lost 2 pounds."
> Nurse: "Congratulations on the weight you have lost. It can be very difficult to lose weight."

Patient: "That is for sure. I don't understand it. I kept up with my exercise routine, so I should have continued losing weight. The only thing I can think of that could have been the problem was that I ate out more since my wife has been working longer hours."

Nurse: "Your wife is the one who primarily cooks the meals."

Patient: "Yes. I know how to cook, but it is easier to eat out. I know I need to eat better."

Nurse: Silence

Patient: "I have been thinking about ways to eat better. Dinner is the problem because I am hungry after work and I don't have the energy or desire to cook a meal."

Nurse: "You are considering the possibilities. What do you think is your next step?"

Patient: "Well, I thought I'd go shopping and buy some things that can be made ahead of time, so my wife can eat healthier, also."

This interaction is similar to the previous scenario when it is initiated, but each encounter took a different path. In the first encounter the patient accomplished the original goal and continues with the present goal but changes the process or plan for how to accomplish that goal. In the second encounter the patient did not accomplish the original goal of weight loss through exercise. He chose to continue with the current goal of weight loss, address the barriers, and create a new goal of incorporating healthy nutrition into his daily routine. Another possible scenario could be that the patient is excelling in attaining the goal and shares with the nurse a completely different issue that requires the whole nursing process to start all over again.

SUMMARY

Motivational interviewing fits very well into the basics of nursing practice, which include the use of therapeutic communication and the nursing process. From these basics of nursing we can expand our practice to incorporate behavior change into our daily routine. With proper communication the patient and nurse establish a rapport to work together toward a common goal—the well-being of our patients.

REFERENCES

Bastable, S. (2006). *Essentials of patient education.* Sudbury, MA: Jones and Bartlett.

Bolton, R. (1979). *People skills: How to assert yourself, listen to others, and resolve conflicts.* New York: Simon & Schuster.

Botelho, R. (2004). *Motivational practice: Promoting healthy habits and self care of chronic diseases.* Rochester, NY: MHH Publications.

Ellis, J. R., Nowlis, E., & Bentz, P. (1992). *Modules for basic nursing skills* (vol. 1, 5th ed.). Philadelphia: J.B. Lippincott.

Haber, J., McMahon, A. L., Price-Hoskins, P., & Sileau, B. F. (1992). *Comprehensive psychiatric nursing* (4th ed.). St. Louis, MO: Mosby Year Book.

Miller, W., & Rollnick, S. (2002). *Motivational interviewing: Preparing people for change* (2nd ed.). New York: The Guilford Press.

Miller, W., & Rollnick, S. (2003). The philosophy behind motivational interviewing. Retrieved September 25, 2008, from http://motivationalinterview.org/clinical/whatismi.html

Pender, N., Murdaugh, C. L., & Parsons, M. (2002). *Health promotion in nursing practice* (4th ed.). Upper Saddle River, New Jersey: Prentice Hall.

Roberts, S. (2005). *Communication for health action: Motivating change* (3rd ed.). The Permanente Medical Group.

Rollnick, S., Mason, P., & Butler, C. (1999). *Health behavior change: A guide for practitioners.* Edinburgh: Churchill Livingstone.

Rollnick, S., Miller, W. R., & Butler, C. C. (2008). *Motivational interviewing in health care: Helping patients change behavior.* New York: The Guilford Press.

Schenk, S., & Hartley, K. (2002). Nurse coach: Healthcare resource for this millennium. *Nursing Forum, 37*(3), 14–20.

Stone, D., Patton, B., & Heen, S. (1999). *Difficult conversations: How to discuss what matters most.* New York: Penguin.

Welch, M. (2005). Pivotal moments in the therapeutic relationship. *International Journal of Mental Health Nursing, 14,* 161–165.

CHAPTER 3

Motivational Interviewing as Evidence-Based Practice

———— OBJECTIVES ————

After completing this chapter, the reader will be able to

1. Discuss the importance of research in evidence-based practice.
2. Describe how motivational interviewing can help reach the goals set forth in Healthy People 2010.
3. Differentiate between MISC and MITI.
4. State at least three general guidelines used in evaluating effective use of motivational interviewing.
5. Compare and contrast the three landmark studies.
6. List at least three areas where research has shown motivational interviewing to be of some benefit.

———— KEY TERMS ————

Adaptations of motivational
   interviewing (AMI)
Brief motivational interventions
Chronic care model
Healthy People 2010
Home-based chronic care model
Motivational enhancement therapy
   (MET)

Medication interest model
Motivational interviewing skill code
   (MISC)
Motivational interviewing treatment
   integrity (MITI)
Project CARES
Project COMBINE
Project MATCH

IMPORTANCE OF RESEARCH

Building a profession on solid scientific evidence requires research studies. Nursing prides itself on evidence-based practice. Proving that a practice is effective supports what we are doing. This research also provides us with information that helps to change areas that are ineffective. The future of our profession is shaped by research.

Healthy People 2010 is a national effort to improve the nation's overall health. This initiative was created to provide focus to areas that need improvement in health promotion. These goals are to be met by the year 2010, and the next initiative for 2020 will then be put into motion. The leading health indicators for reaching the present goals are physical activity, overweight and obesity, tobacco use, substance abuse, responsible sexual behavior, mental health, injury and violence, environmental quality, immunization, and access to health care. These health indicators "were selected on the basis of their ability to motivate action, the availability of data to measure progress, and their importance as public health issues" (healthypeople.gov/LHI/lhiwhat.htm). The use of motivational interviewing can only enhance our success in reaching the health promotion goals set out for us. These leading health indicators are highly dependent upon changing behaviors.

Healthy People 2010 helps shape the focus for our practice based on statistical data, but we also need a method of practice to accomplish those goals that is based on scientific research. Many studies have been done to establish that motivational interviewing is effective in a wide range of areas. The CINAHL and Medline databases were searched for research studies on motivational interviewing in nursing practice, specifically. The result of this search revealed that some were about the use in nursing practice, but most were related to mental health professions or general health professions. We can rationalize that nurses can use this method of behavior change for all areas shown to be effective up to this point, but clearly more research needs to be done in all areas of nursing practice to stake a claim in this innovative method of promoting behavior change.

HOW WE EVALUATE THE USE OF MOTIVATIONAL INTERVIEWING

In this section we look at individual research studies and meta-analyses of various studies. There are randomized and nonrandomized control studies. Many studies really look at **adaptations of motivational interviewing (AMIs)**, which are changes to motivational interviewing techniques or brief interventions using motivational interviewing tactics. There are two main tools to measure the accuracy of motivational interviewing skills to ensure fidelity of motivational interviewing in the field of research: the **motivational interviewing skill code (MISC)** version 2.1 and **motivational interviewing treatment integrity (MITI)** version 3.0. "The MISC gathers information to help understand the mechanisms by which Motivational Interviewing works, and captures both counselor and client behaviors as well as ratings of the interaction" (Breger, DeFrancesco, & Elliot, 2005, p. 14). This tool has a variety of codes for both the client and the counselor and is used by listening and coding the interaction two times. Each area is rated on a seven-point Likert scale. The ratings for the global counselor ratings are based on an entire interaction between the healthcare professional and client. The global client ratings are based on a portion of the interaction where the client is at the highest point of self-exploration (Miller, Moyers, Ernst, & Amrhein, 2008) (Figure 3-1). "The MITI captures only counselor behaviors and measures the fidelity of the interaction to Motivational Interviewing" (Breger et al., 2005, p. 14). This coding system is simpler to use with fewer areas to rate (Figure 3-2).

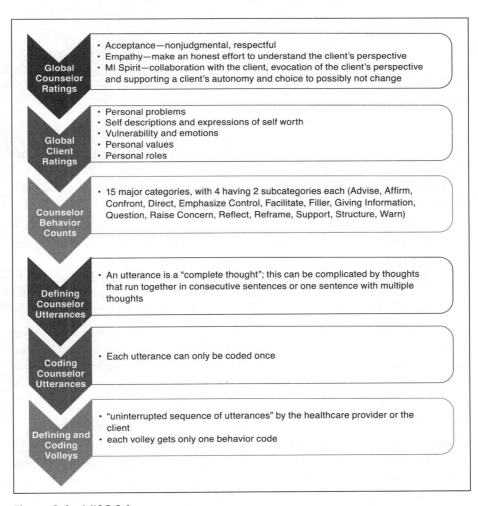

Figure 3-1   MISC 2.1

Source: Adapted from Miller, W., et al., 2008.

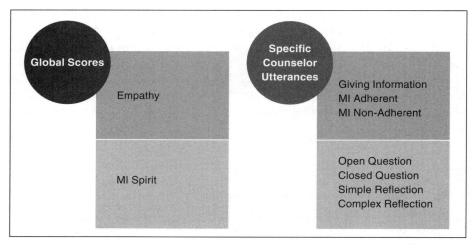

Figure 3-2   MITI 3.0

Source: Adapted from Breger et al., 2005.

For the sake of simplicity general guidelines can be followed and easily assessed for effectiveness, but these guidelines are not as intensive as that needed for scientific research. The guidelines can be used in general practice for skill evaluation and are as follows (Miller & Rollnick, 2002):

- Talk less than the client
- There should be two to three reflections to every one question asked by the provider.
- Open questions to closed questions should be a ratio of 2:1.
- Less than one-half of reflections should be simple restatements or rephrasing and more than one-half should be more complex reflections

Although these tools are available, they are not always noted to have been used in the research studies. The MITI is still in its development but can be used in studies now. Having these scales and coding tools will only increase the validity of upcoming research studies.

RESEARCH STUDIES REVIEWED

There are multiple review articles about studies that have been done to support the effectiveness of motivational interviewing. Of the countless studies done, only a few are particularly important in the growth of motivational interviewing. These landmark studies include **Project MATCH**, **Project COMBINE**, and **Project CARES**. Additional individual studies are also reviewed here to reinforce the importance of scientific evidence that motivational interviewing can, in fact, improve nursing practice.

Meta-Analysis of Research Studies

In this section we look at five groups of people who have performed a meta-analysis on studies done on the effectiveness of motivational interviewing. These articles were published between 2001 and 2005. Greater than 200 studies were reviewed in total. Many studies have been done with the use of AMIs, and this may actually be beneficial because often there is not enough time to do more than a brief intervention, and this is more realistic for our daily practice.

The first review focused on 72 randomized controlled studies (Rubak, Sandbaek, Lauritzen, & Christensen, 2005). The studies included had to clearly state that motivational interviewing was used as it was defined by Stephen Rollnick and William Miller. Most of the encounters in these studies were one-on-one and lasted about 1 hour. The number of encounters was on average one, two, or more than five. Psychologists were the primary providers, but it was noted that the educational background did not impact the effect of motivational interviewing, and no findings suggested that nurses would be any less effective in using this tool for behavior change. Most of the studies focused on alcohol abuse but also looked at other areas, such as diabetes, weight loss, physical activity, and asthma. Motivational interviewing showed effectiveness regardless if the focus was on psychological or physiological issues. Being able to transfer these skills into a variety of areas ensures that this method can be used in all areas of practice, and the possibilities are endless (Rubak et al., 2005).

The second review article included 30 randomized controlled clinical studies (Burke, Arkowitz, & Menchola, 2003). The difference between this and the previous review is that these studies looked at the effectiveness of AMIs. There was a significant difference among the studies of the length of each session and the length of the follow-up period. The average session of AMI was 99 treatment minutes. The average length for follow-up was 18 weeks. Overall, AMIs were found to be effective in areas of drugs, alcohol, diet, and exercise. The studies reviewed were not able to support effectiveness of AMIs in areas of smoking cessation and HIV risk behaviors. This may come down to simple numbers. There were more studies reviewed in the areas that were found to be effectively treated with AMI. It was interesting to note that AMI cannot only improve a target symptom, such as alcohol abuse, but can also reach beyond and positively affect other areas in one's life (Burke et al., 2003).

Another meta-analysis reviewed 29 studies (Dunn, Deroo, & Rivara, 2001). These studies were randomized trials of both motivational interviewing and

AMIs. It was not always clear which form of treatment was used. The focus of the studies included substance abuse, smoking, HIV risk, and diet/exercise. The findings supported effectiveness of motivational interviewing in the area of substance abuse, regardless of who performed the treatment. This factor supports the use of motivational interviewing in nursing practice (Dunn et al., 2001).

There were several commentaries about this particular review article from experts, such as Stephen Rollnick and William Miller. Rollnick (2001) noted that AMIs were more often used than motivational interviewing tactics. These studies were not all clear about how motivational interviewing or AMIs were used and leaves to question if the methods were closely enough related to motivational interviewing to form accurate results. He also looked at training and provider perspective. Providers need proper training and may require counseling to help change their individual behavior. As healthcare professionals, we have taken on a paternalistic role with our patients and need to be consistent in our approach to coexist with our patients. The client-centered approach is primary to motivational interviewing (Rollnick, 2001).

Miller (2001) noted the fact that tools, such as the MITI and MISC, for evaluating motivational interviewing skills were not fully developed at the time these studies were conducted and are in development even at this time. He stated that more studies could have been included in the review and that some studies should not have been excluded because of a lack of a monitoring system. It is not clear what needs to be monitored because little is known about the actual mechanisms of motivational interviewing that make this form of treatment effective. He recognized that it is challenging to evaluate a style of counseling, but direct monitoring should be the gold standard. Of special note, Dunn et al. (2001) found that motivational interviewing was effective when used versus no treatment, but there was an amplified effect when used along with other forms of treatment. Miller (2001) stated that motivational interviewing may exert a synergistic effect. This is of benefit to the nursing practice because motivational interviewing would be used as an additive tool to the many skills already used in practice (Miller, 2001).

Hettema, Steel, and Miller (2005) reviewed 72 studies, with a majority focusing on alcohol and drug abuse. Other areas looked at smoking, HIV risk, treatment compliance, water purification, diet/exercise, gambling, eating disorders, and relationships. Motivational interviewing was compared with no treatment, specified treatment, typical treatment, and additive treatment. There were certain characteristics of motivational interviewing that had to occur to be included in this review and the average covered was 3.6 of the following characteristics:

- Collaborative
- Client centered
- Nonjudgmental

- Building trust
- Reducing resistance
- Increasing readiness
- Increasing self-efficacy
- Reflective listening
- Increasing discrepancy
- Eliciting change talk
- Exploring ambivalence
- Expressing empathy

The average length of treatment was two sessions, and providers had an average of 10 hours of training. Nurses were included in some of these studies as the provider. Findings were that the effects of motivational interviewing is demonstrated early and diminish over time, unless used with other forms of treatment. They concluded that motivational interviewing not only increases treatment adherence but also treatment retention and staff-perceived motivation. It was also noted that the effects of this treatment decreases over the course of a year, but not necessarily so when motivational interviewing was used in conjunction with other forms of treatment. There was a lot of variability in regards to some factors. The effectiveness of motivational interviewing was not related to any particular type of provider, and treatment process variables had more of an impact. Again, nurses can be just as effective in using motivational interviewing tactics as other providers (Hettema et al., 2005).

In Chapter 16 of their book, Miller and Rollnick (2002) reviewed some of the research behind motivational interviewing. The authors took advantage of the increased number of studies that had accumulated by this time and looked at these studies from both a quantitative and qualitative perspective. From a quantitative perspective, the use of AMIs in the area of alcohol use/abuse is effective. The effectiveness in other areas was less conclusive. They looked at 26 randomized, controlled, clinical studies. All interventions were individual and face-to-face encounters. Interestingly, it was found that AMI can be effective as a one-time treatment as noted in one study where the treatment occurred at a trauma center in hopes to decrease the risk of future injury. The studies did not use motivational interviewing in its true form but rather as AMIs (Miller & Rollnick, 2002).

One to four sessions of AMI was found to be effective in the areas of alcohol and drug addiction. There was also a finding that the AMIs could maintain these effects over time. Again, Miller and Rollnick concluded from the review that AMI is better than no treatment and is at least as effective as other treatments. They found that the effectiveness is not limited to alcohol and drug dependence but extends to other areas, such as diabetes, eating disorders, and hypertension. Ultimately, AMIs have been found to be better than no treatment at all and are equal in efficacy to other forms of treatment. In fact, AMIs can provide a synergistic effect when combined with other treatments (Miller & Rollnick, 2002).

There has clearly been a drive to prove motivational interviewing's worth to healthcare practice. It is important to recognize that nurses play a vital role in helping patients to transform their lives through motivation and empowerment. This can be done effectively by incorporating motivational interviewing into each nurse–patient encounter.

Landmark Studies

It has clearly been established that motivational interviewing or AMIs can be an effective form of treatment in a number of areas. A few landmark studies provide additional insight into how motivational interviewing works and how it can impact certain areas of practice. Project MATCH is a randomized, controlled, multiple site study that compared three different types of treatment for alcohol addiction, including **motivational enhancement therapy (MET)**. MET is an AMI. In this study the 1,726 patients had 12 weeks of treatment and then follow-up for 1 year at 3-month intervals (http://www.niaaa.nih.gov/News Events/NewsReleases/match.htm). One important factor in this study was the use of a feedback approach. The patients were given feedback from the provider using a motivational interviewing style. The MET technique was found to be effective and comparative with the other forms of treatment, such as the 12-step therapy and cognitive behavioral therapy, two other gold standards in alcohol treatment (Miller & Rollnick, 2002).

Project COMBINE is another study that looked at treatment for those with alcohol dependence. There were 1,383 patients randomized for enrollment in this study (http://www.cscc.unc.edu/combine/whowas.htm). This study focused on comparing the use of medical management alone, behavioral therapy alone, and a combination of medical and behavioral management. (This combined behavioral intervention is also referred to as CBI.) The medication naltrexone was found to be effective, alone or in combination with a motivational interviewing technique. The behavioral therapy was found to be just as effective alone or in combination with the naltrexone. In previous studies the motivational interviewing tactics were synergistic with other forms of treatment, but that was not the case in this study. The medication alone, behavioral therapy, and the combination were found to be equally effective (Anton et al., 2006; Miller & Rollnick, 2002).

Project CARES focused on studying smoking cessation. Home health nurses were randomly assigned to provide MET with the feedback being patient's carbon monoxide levels on expiration. There were 98 nurses and 273 patients included in this study. The patients were either provided with MET or standard care according to the Agency for Health Care Policy and Research guidelines for smoking cessation. Follow-up occurred for 12 months after treatment. It was found that MET was more effective in regards to attempts to quit smoking and the number of cigarettes smoked per day. Ultimately, there was a positive effect that extends to the community. This is great progress for the nursing community and its ability to transform the way in which we provide care (Borelli, B. et al., 2005).

These three studies provided us with some very important information about motivational interviewing and what it has to offer nursing practice. Two of these studies proved the benefit of MET and its use of feedback during the intervention. We can see evidence of motivational interviewing effectiveness in areas of chronic illness and in health promotion. If we can reach the masses and empower the people of our communities, we can attain the goals set out for us by Healthy People 2010.

Exploring the Lessons Learned From Research

A variety of research studies can support the use of motivational interviewing in nursing practice. Studies have been done to look at cost savings, which is of great significance during these economic times. Not only is it important to look at the effect of motivational interviewing on patients and their lives, it is also essential to include information about the provider's skills and perspectives. Different environments can produce different results on how effective a treatment may be. A patient can receive treatment in an office, through home health, and via a telephone or computer. Nurses have always focused on the whole person: the physical, social, and emotional. Motivational interviewing provides us with another tool to allow us to continue with our focus.

Cost-Effectiveness

One study that directly addressed the financial aspect of motivational interviewing looked at medication adherence versus long-term complications costs. There are many chronic diseases that require ongoing medication use. Wiegand and Wertheimer (2008) focused on type 2 diabetes. The costs of type 2 diabetes care, yearly medication costs and the total cost of behavioral therapy over a period of 16 years, were calculated. When calculating the costs of complications, they looked at the percentage of patients and the cost for one complication and those with two or more complications. The findings were a potential savings of $23,000 per patient. This is an incredible amount of money that could be used in other areas of health care (Wiegand & Wertheimer, 2008).

The reasons people do not take their medication are important to understand. In a paternalistic practice, we would tell a patient they need to take their medication and, perhaps, give them reasons why they need it. When using a motivational interviewing approach, we would ask what keeps them from taking their medication routinely. Initial questions need to be nonjudgmental to avoid immediate resistance. The following are some possible statements the nurse might say during a conversation with a patient about the topic of medication adherence:

- "Share with me your current medication regimen."
- "You are not able to get into a routine for taking your medication. Something is in your way."
- "Sometimes we know something is meant to be helpful but is very difficult to follow through with."
- "I would be interested to hear what you think would help you to remember to take your medication."
- "I hear you saying that the side effects to the medication are very disturbing to you. You want to get the symptoms of your disease under control, but you feel you are just substituting for other uncomfortable symptoms."
- "You feel good and don't believe you need these medications."
- "Taking medication everyday can be costly. I'm curious if this has been a barrier to you taking your medication."

There are times when our preconceptions cloud our views, making it challenging to go into a motivational interviewing session and leave the patient empowered. A person that does not take his or her medication as prescribed has been thought of as "noncompliant." This gives a negative connotation to a person who may have valid reasons for not being able to follow the recommendations set forth by the healthcare provider. Go into each encounter knowing there is an opportunity to discover who this person is and where he or she comes from and wants to go.

The **medication interest model** uses motivational interviewing to help patients explore the reasons for not taking medication. This model is based on three basic premises:

1. The patient believes there is something wrong.
2. The patient is motivated to improve what is wrong.
3. The patient believes there are more "pros" than "cons" to taking medication.

If a person does not accept that he or she has an illness or problem, that person will not be motivated to treat that problem. Some patients may accept that there is a problem but do not see a benefit in treating it. There may be a desire to try other forms of treatment, or the patient may want more information before he or she commits to a treatment plan. Even if the nurse believes that it should be a clear choice to choose treatment, the patient needs to see the benefits outweigh the consequences to take steps and stick with a course of treatment. As advocates for our patients, we need to remember that we are advocating for them and not for ourselves or our beliefs.

In regards to cost-effectiveness, motivational interviewing can clearly be seen to help with healthcare costs in type 2 diabetes. Medication adherence is an issue in all areas of health care. An assumption is made that this positive impact can be carried into the treatment of other chronic illness care. More research needs to be done to prove this statement.

Provider Skills and Perspectives

Incorporation of motivational interviewing into nursing practice requires training, practice, and feedback. A randomized controlled study was performed to evaluate the provider's skill level on the effectiveness of motivational interviewing. Five counselors provided **brief motivational interventions**, which is an AMI. There were 95 of these interventions performed by the counselors, who had similar training. The sessions were recorded and coded using the MISC. The findings of this study support higher skill levels are more effective overall but that lower skill levels could be effective when the patient is at a high level of ability to change (Gaume, Gmel, Faouzi, & Daeppen, 2009).

A single session of 15 minutes was performed with the experimental group of patients with alcohol dependence and/or abuse. The counselors had specific criteria for that encounter. Follow-up was performed at 12 months. All counselors in this study were master's prepared psychologists with 1 year of clinical experience and one "experienced" nurse. There were no further details to describe the nurse's background, other than all counselors received similar training. The study found significant variability in counselor skills but did not specify where the nurse was on the continuum. Higher skill level is assumed to bring higher efficacy, and this study supported this belief (Gaume et al., 2009).

All the research that supports the use of motivational interviewing is reassuring. Without the support of those providing care to the patients, it is just another tool that becomes rusted. Rash (2008a) explored what some providers really think about this practice. A study was done with a goal to decrease alcohol-related events in high-risk college students, and Rash interviewed the physicians, a family nurse practitioner, and a physician's assistant who participated in that study. Each provider had no previous experience with motivational interviewing and received the same training. It was challenging to change their approach. There were similarities in this new way of interacting with the patient and what they had traditionally used for interviewing techniques. Motivational interviewing has specific steps to take to communicate versus a more general approach of therapeutic communication. Ultimately, Rash found that the providers agreed on the following:

- Motivational interviewing is more successful than a directive approach.
- Motivational interviewing is a more "satisfying" way to interact for both the provider and the patient.
- Motivational interviewing has potential to be a positive adjunct in the college health environment.

Rash (2008a) also reported that the providers are more supportive of AMIs than the unabridged motivational interviewing tactics because of time constraints.

The healthcare provider has an important role in creating a home for motivational interviewing in practice. Advanced motivational interviewing skills are crucial to increasing the effectiveness of this tool that will not only promote behavior change but will empower our patients to take the necessary steps to healthy lifestyles. In Chapter 15, we discuss ways to learn about motivational interviewing and how to increase the skills to properly and effectively use this method. As more providers incorporate motivational interviewing into practice, more research can be done to support what some providers have already found, a successful and rewarding way to interact with patients and change behaviors (Rash, 2008a).

Motivational Interviewing in the Office

Primary and specialty care in the office setting does not always allow for sufficient time to investigate a patient's problems, level of readiness to change and to explore ways in which the patient can go about making changes, should he or she be ready. As we have seen from the research, time constraints can be solved by use of AMIs. Even short interactions of 15 minutes can make a difference. This goes along with how we often handle patient education. Often, information is provided in small amounts over a period of time. Consider each encounter a stepping stone toward empowerment and behavior change. It is amazing how much can actually be accomplished when we have adequate tools.

Simmons, Baker, Schaefer, Miller, and Anders (2009) addressed the need for brief interventions that are easy to learn and support a collaborative relationship between patient and provider. The first step is for the patient to create a health goal with the support of the provider. This can be challenging if the patient does not perceive a problem as noted in a previous study. Once the health goal is determined, the provider and patient can then work together to create a plan. The authors found a study that evaluated the amount of time it takes for the planning stage. This particular study found the average time to be 6.9 minutes with a minimum of 1 minute and a maximum of 20 minutes. In follow-up, evaluation of the patient's progress can occur, and if there are problems, reassessment and goal setting would have to reoccur (Simmons et al., 2009). Time is always a factor, and as we become more proficient with motivational interviewing skills, we can have effective interactions in short periods of time.

Time is limited in the office setting. A patient is likely to have only 15 minutes or less with the provider and that includes an exam. There are many areas of our lives that we could change to decrease our risks for illness, improve our current health status, and prevent long-term complications of current illnesses. It is overwhelming to think about the importance of addressing these issues with our patients when we have such limited time to interact with them. Prevention of obesity and type 2 diabetes has been at the forefront of nursing and all other healthcare professions. Two studies looked at these areas of concern.

The first study evaluated a lifestyle program that was provided by nurse practitioners (Whittemore et al., 2009). The program was planned for a 6-month period, but the average length of the program lasted 9.3 months. Training was more intense for the nurse practitioners providing behavioral therapy in the lifestyle program. The lifestyle program consisted of six in-person sessions and five telephone sessions over 6 months. The in-person sessions lasted 20 minutes. Based on the amount of weight loss and the decrease in risk of type 2 diabetes, this study found the intervention to be "modestly" effective (Whittemore et al., 2009).

Pediatricians and nutritionists provided motivational interviewing in a nonrandomized clinical trial to prevent childhood obesity. The second study looked at children between the ages of 3 and 7 with a body mass index between the 85th and 95th percentiles or with parents with a body mass index of 30 or greater (Schwartz et al., 2007). One group received one motivational interviewing session and the other group received two sessions. At the 6-month follow-up there was a notable decrease in body mass index profiles in each of the groups, but no group showed superior results. One significant finding was that 94% of the parents found the intervention helpful to consider making changes in the family's eating habits. The authors concluded that motivational interviewing in the office setting can be a positive influence on preventing childhood obesity (Schwartz et al., 2007).

More research can support the use of motivational interviewing in the office setting. It is obvious from these studies, however, that there is definite potential to have a positive impact on health prevention.

Home Health Care

We have already seen from Project CARES that motivational interviewing can be used in the home health arena. As many home health nurses know, most care for these patients revolves around their chronic care issues. Motivational interviewing is a useful tool to promote behavior change for those with chronic illness. Suter and coworkers (2008) highlighted the importance of self-management and our role in supporting the patient to be more proactive in his or her care. Disease management is a process that helps to empower patients to make choices, promote self-management, and prevent long-term complications (Suter et al., 2008).

Often, the provider focuses on the acute issues and the chronic health issues are not adequately addressed. The home health providers work in conjunction with the primary provider to meet the patients' variable needs. Suter et al. (2008) looked at two care models used in chronic care. The **chronic care model** helps guide how we care for patients with chronic illness. As previously stated, home health is one environment in which chronic care needs can be more effectively addressed. The second model, the **home-based chronic care model**, builds on the previous model. Specific aspects of these models are not provided in detail. The home environment is conducive to enhanced disease management and is also cost-effective. The arguments for care to be provided in the home environment include but are not limited to a more comfortable atmosphere to build trust, a better understanding of the patient's abilities and resources, and insight to barriers that may prevent the patient from being able to properly self-manage (Suter et al., 2008).

As we go forward in a wavering economy, the importance of providing effective care in a cost-effective manner will only increase. Our role, as nurses in the home health environment, will evolve to better provide care to those with chronic illness. Motivational interviewing is one of many tools that will help us to improve our practice during this time of evolution.

Telephonic Interventions

Despite the benefit of face-to-face interactions between the nurse and patient, telephone-based practice is growing. Disease management programs are being provided through health insurance companies, employers, and health promotion initiatives. One article focused on motivational interviewing for diabetes management, the other on a smoking cessation program.

Dale, Caramlau, Sturt, Friede, and Walker (2009) provided a new perspective on the use of motivational interviewing. This study tested trial design issues that could occur when evaluating effectiveness of the telephone intervention's ability to promote self-efficacy and the impact on self-efficacy and clinical outcomes. Peer support persons and diabetes specialty nurses performed the telephone interaction with the patients. A total of 231 patients were a part of this study. The interactions occurred over a 6-month period of time. The patients were very accepting of the program, but the support provided by the diabetes specialty nurses was more valued than that of the peer supporters. There was not a significant change in outcome measures. The authors reported that motivational interviewing can be used telephonically with people with poorly controlled type 2 diabetes but may not be effective for all patients (Dale et al., 2009). This is the case with all treatment modalities. Part of the nurse's role is to help identify what tools benefit the patient most. Motivational interviewing is one of those tools that offers great benefit to many but not all.

Patten and colleagues (2008) evaluated the effectiveness of a telephone-based intervention that provided treatment to support persons who desired to help someone quit smoking. This study did not specifically report use of motivational interviewing. It was based on the social cognitive–based model of health behavior change. The intervention sought to increase the support person's motivation level to change his or her own behaviors. Promotion of self-efficacy was another goal. The use of positive reinforcement was also an important factor. There were six counseling sessions, and written material was provided. There were 10 support persons receiving treatment and 4 counselors, who were Mayo Clinic Tobacco Quitline staff. They all received the same amount of training. The result of this study was primarily attaining information to revise the treatment protocol to enhance effectiveness for a randomized clinical study (Patten et al., 2008).

Telephone interventions have become more utilized as a practical environment. This method can reach those who are disabled or elderly and have difficulty leaving the home. This treatment modality can work very well for many people but may not be the best form of treatment for all people. Motivational interviewing tactics can be effective telephonically, as well as face-to-face. There may even be a benefit for those who feel more comfortable opening up when they cannot visually connect with the provider. More research needs to be done to help guide the future of telephonic interventions using motivational interviewing.

World Wide Web

Despite the advances in technology, it is difficult to imagine how we, as nurses and healthcare providers, can use motivational interviewing to promote behavior change via the computer. Finfgeld-Connett and Madsen (2008) looked at a form of alcohol treatment for women in Missouri who had qualified to participate in this study who were then randomized to standard treatment or the Web-based treatment. The treatment plan was developed based on a variety of theories and models, including motivational interviewing. Information was available, in addition to bulletin boards and chat functions for the Web-based treatment group. The other group received information in hard copy form and was allowed to contact the researcher with any questions but did not have capability of interacting with other participants. Follow-up was at 3 months. There were no significant findings between the treatment groups. Thus the Web-based intervention is just as effective as traditional treatment methods. This form of treatment has the potential to reach the masses in a cost-effective manner (Finfgeld-Connett & Madsen, 2008).

Rash (2008b) evaluated nurses in a study where students were able to participate in an online chat room tool that allowed them to role play a brief intervention. The students were graded on their attempts at motivational interviewing skills. The students reported the need to practice these skills to master them and become proficient. The students were able to see various benefits of motivational interviewing, including the potential to support behavior change and decrease patient resistance. The online chat feature was found to be superior to reading material alone. Having the ability to interact online, using motivational interviewing, is one more arena where we can reach our patients to promote self-efficacy and behavior change (Rash, 2008b).

SUMMARY

Motivational interviewing has earned its title as evidence-based practice. The studies reviewed here are only a fraction of the research that supports this method of promoting behavior change. As with all treatment modalities, continuing research will help with the ongoing development of this promising tool for practice and reinforce the effectiveness of these tactics. Several meta-analyses have been performed and published to provide a quick review of how motivational interviewing can be an effective tool in health care. Landmark studies provide a basis from which to compare or build on other research. With the present availability of rating tools, such as the MITI and MISC, we can now look for these tools to be used more in research to reinforce the provider's abilities to perform motivational interviewing with skill and proficiency.

We also looked at how motivational interviewing can be a cost-effective tool that can be used in a variety of settings. Students of this form of treatment and providers who have practiced this skill have given praise to the level of effectiveness in being patient friendly and in promoting behavior change and self-efficacy. As we move forward into a questionable future, the need to focus on health promotion and self-management will only expand. With motivational interviewing we can move into the future with confidence. Nursing practice will be affected, and we will be prepared to face the challenges, armed with motivational interviewing as one of many tools to accomplish our goals.

REFERENCES

Anton, R., O'Malley, S., Ciraulo, D., Cisler, R., Couper, D., Donovan, D., Gastfriend, D., Hosking, J., Johnson, B., Longabaugh, R., Mason, B., Mattson, M., Miller, W., Pettinati, H., Randall, C., Swift, R., Weiss, R., Williams, L., & Zweban, A. (2006). Combined pharmacotherapies and behavioral interventions for alcohol dependence: The COMBINE study: A randomized controlled trial. *Journal of the American Medical Association, 295*(17), 2003–2017.

Borelli, B., Novak, S., Hecht, J., Emmons, K., Papandonatos, G., & Abrams, D. (2005). Home health nurses as a new channel for smoking cessation treatment: Outcomes from Project CARES (Community-Nurse Assisted Research and Education on Smoking). *Preventive Medicine, 41,* 815–821.

Breger, R., DeFrancesco, C., & Elliot, D. (2005). Training coders to use the motivational interviewing treatment integrity coding system. *MINUET, 12*(2), 14–16.

Burke, B., Arkowitz, H., & Menchola, M. (2003). The efficacy of motivational interviewing: A meta-analysis of controlled clinical trials. *Journal of Consulting and Clinical Psychology, 71*(5), 843–861.

Dale, J., Caramlau, I., Sturt, J., Friede, T., & Walker, R. (2009). Telephone peer-delivered intervention for diabetes motivation and support: The telecare exploratory RCT. *Patient Education and Counseling, 75,* 91–98.

Dunn, C., Deroo, L., & Rivara, F. P. (2001). The use of brief interventions adapted from motivational interviewing across behavioral domains: A systematic review. *Addiction, 96*(12), 1725–1742.

Finfgeld-Connett, D., & Madsen, R. (2008). Web-based treatment of alcohol problems among rural women results of a randomized pilot investigation. *Journal of Psychosocial Nursing and Mental Health Services, 46*(9), 46–53.

Gaume, J., Gmel, G., Faouzi, M., & Daeppen, J. (2009). Counselor skill influences outcomes of brief motivational interventions. *Journal of Substance Abuse Treatment, 37*(2), 151–159.

Hettema, J., Steel, J., & Miller, W. (2005). A meta-analysis of research on motivational interviewing treatment effectiveness (MARMITE). *Annual Review of Clinical Psychology, 1,* 91–111.

Miller, W. (2001). When is it motivational interviewing? *Addiction, 96,* 1770–1772.

Miller, W., Moyers, T., Ernst, D., & Amrhein, P. (2008). *Manual for the motivational interviewing skill code (MISC)* (version 2.1). Center on Alcoholism, Substance Abuse, and Addictions: The University of New Mexico. Retrieved January 8, 2008, from http://casaa.unm.edu/download/misc/pdf

Miller, W., & Rollnick, S. (2002). *Motivational interviewing: Preparing people for change* (2nd ed.). New York: The Guilford Press.

Moyers, T., Martin, T., Manuel, J., Miller, W., & Ernst, D. (2007). *Revised global scales: Motivational interviewing treatment integrity 3.0 (MITI 3.0).* Center on Alcoholism, Substance Abuse, and Addictions: The University of New Mexico. Retrieved January 8, 2008, from http://casaa.unm.edu/download/MITI3.pdf

Patten, C., Petersen, L., Brockman, T., Gerber, T., Offord, K., Ebbert, J., Hughes, C., Decker, P., Beddow, C., Pyan, K., Quigg, S., & Boness, J. (2008). Development of a telephone-based intervention for support persons to help smokers quit. *Psychology, Health & Medicine, 13*(1), 17–28.

Rash, E. (2008a). Clinician's perspectives on motivational interviewing-based brief interventions in college health. *Journal of American College Health, 57*(3), 379–380.

Rash, E. (2008b). Simulating health promotion in an online environment. *Journal of Nursing Education, 47*(11), 515–517.

Rollnick, S. (2001). Enthusiasm, quick fixes and premature controlled trials. *Addiction, 96,* 1769–1770.

Rubak, S., Sandbaek, A., Lauritzen, T., & Christensen, B. (2005). Motivational interviewing: A systematic review and meta-analysis. *British Journal of General Practice, 55*(513), 305–312.

Schwartz, R., Hamre, R., Dietz, W., Wasserman, R., Slora, E., Myers, E., Sullivan, S., Wasserman, R., Slora, E., Myers, E., Sullivan, S., Rockett, H., Thoma, K., Dumitru, G., & Resnicow, K. (2007). Office-based motivational interviewing to prevent childhood obesity: A feasibility study. *Archives of Pediatric & Adolescent Medicine, 161*, 495–501.

Simmons, L., Baker, N., Schaefer, J., Miller, D., & Anders, S. (2009). Activation of patients for successful self-management. *Journal of Ambulatory Care Management, 32*(1), 16–23.

Suter, P., Hennessey, B., Harrison, G., Fagan, M., Norman, B., & Suter, W. (2008). Home-based chronic care: An expanded integrative model for home health professionals. *Home Healthcare Nurse, 26*(4), 222–228.

Whittemore, R., Melkus, G., Wagner, J., Dziura, J., Northrup, V., & Grey, M. (2009). Translating the diabetes prevention program to primary care: A pilot study. *Nursing Research, 58*(1), 2–12.

Wiegand, P., & Wertheimer, A. (2008). An economic evaluation of anticipated costs and savings of a behavior change intervention to enhance medication adherence. *Pharmacy Practice, 6*(2), 68–73.

CHAPTER 4

Challenges in Motivational Interviewing

OBJECTIVES

After completing this chapter, the reader will be able to

1. Identify three traps in motivational interviewing.
2. Discuss ways to avoid traps in motivational interviewing.
3. List three barriers to overcome for successful motivational interviewing.
4. Describe at least three ways to proceed when a barrier is encountered.
5. Demonstrate appropriate use of the commitment ruler.
6. Provide examples of communication techniques.

KEY TERMS

Amplified reflection
Blaming trap
Change talk
Commitment ruler
Confrontation/denial trap
Double-sided reflection
Expert trap
Labeling trap

OARS (open questions, affirming, reflecting and summarizing)
Premature focus trap
Reframing
Rolling with resistance
The righting reflex
Shifting the focus
Simple reflection

MOTIVATIONAL INTERVIEWING TRAPS

As with any process, motivational interviewing presents challenges or traps into which we can fall. There are six traps we can anticipate may occur during an encounter with an unmotivated patient. Here we review each trap and then discuss methods to avoid or get around these traps (Figure 4-1).

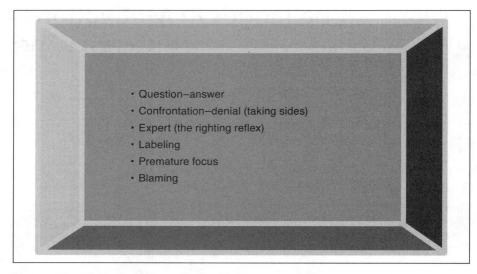

Figure 4-1   Motivational Interviewing Traps

Question–Answer Trap

Asking questions is important to get the answers we need. When seeking to promote behavior change, information about the patient can be helpful to determine which direction the interaction will go. As nurses, we are often hurried to ask quick questions to assess our patients. We have certain information we are seeking. With motivational interviewing the patient holds the answers. The patient has the control.

Motivational interviewing is based on the premise that the patient talks and we provide the feedback and use tactics to help bring out the desire to change. Questions come in different forms. A close-ended question typically results in yes or no responses. An open-ended question allows for the patient to expand on his or her answer and encourages additional information to be shared (Wagner, C., & Conners, W., 2003a). Examples of both types of questions follow:

- Close-ended questions:
  - Are you taking your medication as it is ordered?
  - Have you been exercising routinely?
  - Do you understand what we have talked about?
  - Are you still drinking each day?
  - Will you consider smoking cessation workshops?
- Open-ended questions:
  - What can I help you with today?

- What is the process you go through when you are trying to plan your meals?
- How will you determine your next step?
- When your blood sugar is high, how does that make you feel?
- What would it mean for you to accomplish that goal?

One concern is that the provider takes on a role of being in charge and the patient dutifully answers the questions, one by one. The patient has a passive role, and this goes against the values of motivational interviewing. Also, communication in this manner does not promote exploration of the issues. Ultimately, the goal is to allow the patient to verbalize his or her process of self-exploration and discovery. With proper communication techniques, patients feel comfortable to openly examine where they are, where they want to be, and how they would like to get there. The patients allow us to participate in their journey, and that is important to remember when setting the tone of the interaction. When patients are asked question after question, they will in turn answer each one dutifully. They will less likely explore the issues unless there is a sense of interest from the provider (Wagner, C., & Conners, W., 2003b; Levensky, Forcehimes, O'Donohue, & Beitz, 2007).

One way to avoid this trap is to use more open-ended questions (Wagner, C., & Conners, W., 2003a). This encourages detailed responses from the patient and provides greater insight into the patient as a person with unique challenges. Repetitive open-ended questions can be just as destructive to the patient–provider interaction. The recommendation is to ask "no more than two consecutive questions before offering a reflection" (Levensky et al., 2007, p. 57). Reflecting back to the patient shows the provider is listening and values what the patient has to say, which can only promote a more effective interaction.

Confrontation–Denial Trap

The confrontation–denial trap occurs when the provider presents a case for making changes or reasons for the patient to discontinue his or her current lifestyle. In response, the patient argues that there is no need for change, or the patient may see benefit to staying right where he or she is. This begins a cycle of provider arguments for change and patient support for maintaining status quo (Wagner, C., & Conners, W., 2003b; Levensky et al., 2007). The frustration builds in both the patient and provider, and the chance for a therapeutic encounter is greatly diminished. It is important for the provider to avoid having preconceptions about what patients need to do or what they need not do. The expert is not the provider but, in fact, the patient. When the confrontation–denial cycle occurs, it is a result of the provider acting superior and taking on the expert role. This trap is also known as the "taking sides" trap, where the patient and provider take sides against each other (Miller & Rollnick, 2002).

Providers certainly may have the knowledge to tell people what they should and should not do to improve a health issue, manage symptoms, or what lifestyle changes would benefit a patient. The problem is the provider lacks experience in one area–the patient. We do not live our patients' lives. We do not experience life as they do. We cannot expect patients to simply take our advice and incorporate it into their lifestyle when it may not be realistic for them to carry out. Patients are the experts about what they can and cannot do. They often know what needs to be done but are simply stuck in ambivalence. Patients do not need to hear about what needs to be changed but may need assistance in exploring their ambivalence. The provider takes an important role in helping the patient to move from an ambivalent state into a state of change through motivational interviewing.

This is one of the most challenging traps to avoid. We want to help people and believe we know how people can improve their health. Unsolicited advice is not often welcome. Confrontation, when timed just right, can be used in a positive manner during times when a patient is ready for action (Zerler, 2005). It is difficult for patients to accept recommendations for lifestyle changes if they do not recognize there is a problem or if the information is not conducive to their present lifestyle or what they hope their lifestyle to be. We need to work with the patient and not against them. Following motivational interviewing techniques can help the provider to avoid this trap.

Expert Trap

The "expert trap" is one in which the provider advises the patient without having any information from the patient about what he or she needs, wants, or is ambivalent about (Levensky et al., 2007). This is not to say that the provider cannot share information or offer advice to the patient. By using motivational interviewing, the provider asks permission to share information. During the course of an encounter, we may believe there is information the patient would benefit from. Unfortunately, if the patient is not ready for the information, as demonstrated by resistance or ambivalence, he or she is not likely to follow through with any advice or suggestions. The best time to offer to share information is when the patient is motivated and ready to take some steps toward change.

One concern about this trap is how it can lead the patient to passively accepting the information because the provider is seen as the expert or the one with the knowledge (Wagner, C., & Conners, W., 2003b). This is another trap that prevents the provider and patient from walking hand in hand to explore and discover what the patient is seeking. We can improve this situation by first helping the patient to delve into his or her personal story, goals, and roadblocks. Once the patient has shared a desire to change, the provider can ask permission to also share what may be helpful to his or her process of change. Asking permission shows patients that the provider respects them and honors their space. If they decline, the provider can simply move on. When they accept, the provider has built their confidence in him or her and patients are comfortable with exploring some of their deepest thoughts and emotions with the provider. This type of respectful relationship is what motivational interviewing is all about.

Another name for this trap is the "righting reflex" (Miller & Rollnick, 2002). In the helping professions we strive to make things right, to improve other people's lives. It is our nature to nurture. To let go of that need to right a wrong or fix a problem is a great challenge. We need to accept that the patient may know best how to find an answer or come to a solution. We are there to help guide the way when patients are focused but stray from their path. Otherwise, we are there to simply walk beside them as they search and discover themselves.

Labeling Trap

Too often people are given labels meant to describe a part of who they are. But a person is more than just a label. Many patients resist a diagnosis or a label placed on them, for example, an "alcoholic." Motivational interviewing is intended to deemphasize labels because labels often carry a stigma that people want to avoid (Wagner, & Conners, 2003b). There is no need to place a label on someone to help them move toward changing their behavior. In fact, by labeling someone, the provider is more likely to contribute to resistance and hinder the process. There are many situations to which this could apply, but we never know how a person feels about his or her problem or diagnosis. It is important to be respectful of this trap with every encounter.

Premature-Focus Trap

The premature-focus trap occurs when the provider focuses on a topic before listening to what the patient would like to discuss. The provider determines the focus instead of the patient (Levensky et al., 2007). The patient and provider are working against each other instead of with each other. Motivational interviewing promotes use of open-ended questions and reflections that help to avoid this trap. These tools allow the provider to encourage self-exploration and self-determination throughout the interaction.

Focusing prematurely may occur during the initial phase of the conversation. The provider may assume the focus should be in one area. This trap can also occur later in the conversation when the patient is talking about a certain area of concern. When the provider starts focusing on action when the patient is not ready, the provider has fallen into the trap. Later we discuss some words or phrases that indicate change talk or a readiness to change (See section "Change talk" of this chapter). The conversation between the patient and provider can lead into action once the patient reveals a readiness to take action.

Blaming Trap

There is a desire to blame someone or something for the things that happen in life. A patient may seek to blame someone else for his or her situation or diagnosis (Wagner, & Conners, 2003b). In response, the provider may indicate that the patient is responsible for his or her personal situation. This creates resistance and results in a subtherapeutic encounter. Motivational interviewing adopts a "no fault" policy (Miller & Rollnick, 2002). The focus should be on how the patient is dealing with the problem and what can be done to improve the situation.

Even if the provider does not counter-blame the patient, just allowing the patient to continue a discussion about blame, results in a nontherapeutic encounter. It is a dead end road that needs to be avoided. The best way to address this trap is to tell patients that the concern is about them and how they are feeling about it, how they are dealing with it, or they can correct it. When the patient believes the provider is genuinely concerned and interested in hearing about what he or she needs, the encounter can progress in a positive manner (Rollnick, Mason, & Butler, 1999).

HOW TO AVOID THE TRAPS

Some of the traps sound as though they may be easy to avoid. The provider must have a strong self-awareness. During the course of a conversation, we can easily fall into one or several of these traps. Using silence as a motivational interviewing tool is often difficult. But silence is a powerful tool. During the silence it is a good time to reflect on how we have contributed to where the conversation is at that moment (Rollnick, Miller, & Butler, 2008). It is important to reflect on any display of the expert role, forcing the focus of the encounter or asking too many questions, and controlling the conversation. Silence allows the patient to also reflect and take the next step in the encounter. This helps them to focus. Once the patient can share which direction he or she would like to go, the provider can then refocus and tend to the immediate conversation. It is human nature to want to fill the spaces of silence in a conversation. This takes strong self-restraint for some people.

Recognizing certain patient behaviors also helps in avoiding the traps. When the patient becomes defensive, it is a clue that the provider has said something or conveyed something that the patient wants to avoid. Perhaps the patient does not want to discuss why he or she isn't taking medication because the patient cannot afford it. When the provider asks about the medication, the patient may get defensive. Another scenario is the patient avoiding the topic. When this occurs, the provider may be too direct during the conversation. The patient should be determining the topic of the conversation with the provider, not the provider making that decision. Paying close attention to the patient's statements, facial expressions, tone of voice, and body language can help to identify points where reevaluation needs to occur.

BARRIERS TO EFFECTIVE MOTIVATIONAL INTERVIEWING

There are six barriers to effective motivational interviewing. Resistance occurs when the patient builds a wall between him- or herself and the provider. The patient clearly does not want to proceed any further at the time he or she is resisting. Another barrier is ambivalence. Patient ambivalence is expected and is the basis of motivational interviewing. Getting to the point of ambivalence can be a difficult journey from a state of resistance. Identifying change talk can also prove to be a barrier. It can be difficult to pinpoint the moment when the patient is ready to move forward to a state of action. Not only can the provider's ambivalence interfere, but personal values can also be a barrier. Lack of commitment from the patient is another barrier that can be difficult to overcome. When the provider does not use effective therapeutic communication skills, motivational interviewing will not be successful and behavior change will not occur.

Resistance

There are many reasons a person feels resistant. There could be fear, anger, confusion, lack of understanding, or a lack of self-efficacy. Whatever the reason for the resistance, the provider needs to be in tune with any signals the patient may exhibit that may indicate resistance (Miller & Rollnick, 2002), such as

- Not contributing to the conversation
- Avoidance
- Arguing
- Interrupting
- Denying
- Frequently changing the subject
- Focusing on unimportant issues

Once resistance is recognized, the provider must be able to change the direction of the conversation. The provider must learn to "roll with resistance." This can actually be a positive force if approached in the correct manner. Allow the patient to explore his or her resistance. The provider can use this as a turning point in the conversation. When the patient states he or she sees no harm in being anorexic, the provider may want to provide information about how this is harmful. To roll with resistance, the provider needs to accept that this is where the patient is right now. Helping the patient explore why it is not harmful or how it benefits the patient, helps him or her feel the provider is empathetic. This is the cornerstone of motivational interviewing. "The patient must be the primary source of answers and solutions and the provider must invite, not impose, new perspectives" (Levensky et al., 2007, p. 53).

Ambivalence

Ambivalence is when there are two contradictory perspectives. It is a struggle about where patients are and where they want to be. The patient sees positive and negative aspects of changing and staying the same. Although they see the benefits and detriments to specific behaviors, it is difficult to move in one direction or the other. According to Miller and Rollnick (2002), ambivalence is a state of decisional balance, where the costs and benefits are weighted on each side of the conflict. Although some people are aware of their own ambivalence, not everyone has that self-awareness. This makes the provider's role even more challenging.

The role of the provider is to elicit information from patients that clarifies their ambivalence (Rollnick et al., 2008). With the use of motivational interviewing tools, the provider can promote an open conversation about why the patient is struggling and hanging in the balance. With the use of proper interviewing techniques, the provider can evoke a discussion about the conflict within the patient.

Consider a patient who is examining her excessive exercise as part of her eating disorder. The patient recognizes that exercise is beneficial in many ways but does not want to give up exercise because it is good for her heart and she feels good when she exercises. She is also recognizing that exercising all the time is interfering with her relationship with her family. She is ambivalent. The provider could force the focus to be about the unhealthy part of the exercising, but this would prove to be detrimental (premature-focus trap). With proper use of open-ended questions and reflective listening, the patient will often move to a state of action. The goal is to help the patient travel through stages of resistance and ambivalence and into a state of change.

As a provider, we can have ambivalence too. We must set aside our personal conflicts and values to support a therapeutic atmosphere in which the patient can progress. When our own ambivalence is obvious, it will only prove to build a barrier between the patient and provider. Maintaining objective perspective and nonjudgmental interaction is important for advancement from ambivalence to commitment to change.

Change Talk

The ability to identify change talk is imperative. A patient may not always be clear that he or she is ready to make a change. Rollnick et al. (1999) identified six types of change talk: desire, ability, reasons, need, commitment, and taking steps. Initially, the acronym DARN was used to represent the first four kinds of change talk. Later, commitment was added to the list and was referred to as DARN-C. This acronym is still in the literature, despite the addition of "taking steps" to the list (Rollnick et al., 1999).

Desire

This type of change talk reflects a desire to make a change. This occurs when the patient is no longer comfortable with status quo. They are looking to improve and the signs may be subtle. A simple statement such as "I wish my blood pressure would come down" indicates that they may be interested in talking with the provider about ways to improve the blood pressure. This would be a perfect opportunity to inquire about how they would like to go about making changes to decrease the blood pressure. If they are not sure how it can be done, the provider can ask permission to share some information that may assist them in taking steps toward their goal. There are other phrases that indicate a desire to change (Rollnick et al., 2008):

- "I want to . . ."
- "I would like to . . ."
- "I wish . . ."

Ability

Ability is what the patient feels he or she is capable of accomplishing. You will hear statements beginning with "I could," "I can," "I think I can," or "I might be able to" (Rollnick et al., 2008). When this is heard in the conversation, the patient is exhibiting change talk. Take a look at the following example:

Patient: "I have thought about what I can do to improve my overall health."

Nurse: "You have put some thought into your health and what you feel you could accomplish in taking steps toward improvement."

Patient: "Yes. I can start by watching what I eat. I tend to snack a lot and I love to eat out! I think I'll try to eat out only once a month."

At this point the patient is ready to make a commitment. The provider's role is to gently guide the patient to making that commitment. Ways to provide that guidance are discussed throughout this text.

Reasons

Reasons are "specific arguments for change" (Rollnick et al., 2008). In this case there are no specific words or phrases to provide clues. Active listening is necessary to detect this kind of change talk. The patient presents you with a case for why change would be good. The following are some examples of how it may play out in conversation:

1. Nurse: "To summarize, we have talked about the possible need for a liver transplant, what that means for you and your family and what you feel has contributed to you being where you are today."

   Patient: "That's correct. I need to stop drinking alcohol all together so I can stop any further damage and be more likely to get a new liver, if I need one someday."

   (In this example, the patient has a reason to stop drinking.)

2. Patient: "I am looking for an easier life. I have spent the past 20 years having sex with different partners and I don't want to take the risks anymore. I don't want to feel used anymore."

   Nurse: "You deserve to be treated better than that."

   Patient: "I think so. I am finally ready to make some much needed changes in my life."

   (This patient wants to improve her self-worth and stop living a risky lifestyle.)

3. Nurse: "You said earlier that you know what needs to be done. You recognize there are some challenges to get you where you would like to be and not sure you are able to face those challenges."

   Patient: "That is true. Mostly, I'm afraid of failing and I'm afraid of change. Despite those fears, I know that I can't reach my goal if I don't try. And if nothing else, I need to feel better physically and this is the only way I see how right now."

   (There is recognition of the difficulties in reaching their goal, but they can specify a reason to still make changes.)

Change is never easy but when a change is to be made, there is always a reason why that change should occur.

Need

This kind of change talk occurs when patients believe they have to make a change. There is not always a desire to change, but at times there is a sense that there is no choice and a change is necessary. The words that trigger the provider to recognize this form of change talk are "need," "have to," "got to," "should," "ought," and "must" (Rollnick et al., 2008). The following examples are needs statements:

- "I need a break. I like to use my free time to relax and get high. There must be other ways for me to have some time for me."
- "I really have to make another appointment with the specialist."
- "I've got to stop stressing about the past and start living for the future."
- "I should talk with my family so they can understand where I am at right now."
- "I ought to really try hard to take my medication daily because it does make me feel better."
- "I must get my life in order. So much time has been lost in a drunken haze."

Statements such as these require intervention to take advantage of this moment of clarity when the patient can see that something needs to be done.

Commitment

Commitment is actually a type of change talk. This comes when the patient is beyond discussing the pros and cons of making a change. They may come to you all ready for change and the transition to commitment is a simpler process. Commitment can come in different levels. In the most obvious scenario, the patient states, "I will . . ." In a less obvious expression, the patient may use phrases such as "I promise . . .," "I am ready to . . .," I intend to . . .," "I will consider it," "I hope to . . .," or "I will try to . . ." (Rollnick et al., 2008).

There may not always be a strong level of commitment uttered. It is important to encourage even the lowest levels of commitment, to help the patient along the continuum from a low level of commitment to a high level of commitment. Any window of opportunity to help a person progress toward change should be fostered.

Taking Steps

During the first encounter you may hear the patient state that some action has already been taken toward accomplishing a goal. Rollnick et al. (2008) stated that you are more likely to encounter this form of change talk during subsequent encounters. Although the patient is already in the midst of change, these statements are important. It allows an opportunity for the provider to offer praise for all that has been accomplished. When recognizing that taking steps is not easy, the provider reinforces the efforts that are made, and this can be encouraging to the patient to see the positive effects and continue on his or her path. The following phrases indicate an action has occurred:

- "I tried . . ."
- "I attempted . . ."
- "I am working toward . . ."
- "I have been doing it . . ."
- "I accomplished . . ."

Patients can express a process of change in many other ways. Because change occurs with road blocks, the provider must help the patient to prepare for how to maintain the change or even move forward to reach a larger goal that is accomplished in stages. The process is part of a cycle. It is essential for the provider to be aware and on the lookout for any statements that may indicate change is on the horizon or already occurring.

Personal Values

A provider's personal values may conflict with the patient's personal values. This certainly can be a barrier when the provider struggles with remaining nonjudgmental. Miller (2004) believed there is no such thing as "value-free" therapy. Throughout our interactions with patients, we must make decisions about what direction to take and what to say at certain times, and all of this is affected by our personal values (Miller, 2004). Patients and providers both come to an interaction with traits that can and will affect the encounter. According to Botelho (2004), the following patient and provider factors impact the outcome of a clinical encounter:

- Assumptions
- Roles
- Attitudes
- Beliefs
- Values
- Culture

Both Miller and Botelho recognized that personal values are impossible to leave behind when interacting with a patient. We bring all of who we are to each interaction. Self-awareness is essential, but even when the provider has a strong sense of self-awareness, there may need to be further examination of the provider's skills to ensure personal values are helping and not hindering the process.

Imposition of the provider's values onto the patient becomes an ethical issue. Miller (2004), along with Stephen Rollnick, addressed this issue. They "specifically argued that ethical complexities increase with each of five conditions: (1) the counselor has an opinion as to the desirable outcome; (2) the aspirations of client and counselor differ; (3) the counselor has an investment in a particular outcome; (4) the counselor's personal investment potentially conflicts with the client's best interests, and (5) the counselor has coercive power to influence the direction that the client takes"(Miller, 2004, p. 19).

In many situations the counselor may have personal opinions about a topic of conversation. Often, we become emotionally invested in our patients over a period of time and begin to believe we know what is best for them. Despite our personal convictions, it is important to remain objective and not impose our belief system onto the patient as much as possible. For example, a patient has multiple health issues due to poorly controlled diabetes. The provider may have witnessed a loved one suffer from a similar situation. The provider, without realizing it, could impose his or her personal beliefs about the importance of strictly controlling the diabetes to prevent an untimely death. The interaction will likely be one filled with premature-focus and expert traps and/or frequent signs of patient resistance.

In addition to the provider's personal values, we also must be aware of the values shared by a clinic or program. Some clinics do not clearly state their beliefs, and patients may not realize they are working with a person or group of persons that do not share the same value system. For example, there are many places a pregnant teenager can go for care and options. It is important that the teenager be provided with all options to make an informed decision. One problem noted by Miller (2004) was that "sometimes a program's value stance is apparent from its name and literature, and sometimes it is not." This can contribute to a difference between patient and provider aspirations from the onset.

Lack of Commitment

Reaching a point of commitment can be quite challenging. When the patient begins to demonstrate a desire to change, the provider's role is to help take it to the next phase of commitment. One way to do this is to use the "ruler." This is a scale of 0 to 10, with 1 being not ready to commit to change and 10 being at the highest level of commitment. A scale such as this is often used to assist patients in rating their level of pain. In motivational interviewing this "ruler" can be a very useful tool. It is easy to figure out how to deal with a person's response to his or her pain level. They either require pain management or not. With the commitment ruler, it can be a bit more complicated. This tool can be used to assess level of readiness, desire, or commitment (Rollnick et al., 2008).

Use of the ruler is essentially the same. The provider may ask the patient, "On a scale of 0 to 10, with 0 being not at all and 10 being fully committed, where would you rate your level of commitment at this time?" When using this tool there are some questions that can help to further assess commitment, desire, or readiness. A level of 0–3 reflects a lack of commitment. A level of 4–6 demonstrates ambivalence. A level of 7–10 would signify a person is ready to make a commitment (Roberts, 2005).

Understanding what the patient's response means is important. Knowing what to do with the information obtained from the ruler is essential. To further assess a patient's level of readiness, desire, or commitment, several questions can be helpful (Roberts, 2005):

- Straight question: "Why a level 5?"
- Backward question: "Why a level 5 and not a 2?"
- Forward question: "What would it take for you to move from a 5 to a 7 or 8?"

The patient's answer to these questions can provide insight into what it may take to help this patient make a commitment or simply to better understand why he or she is ambivalent.

For the person who is not ready, the provider's role is to raise awareness, elicit change talk, advise and encourage, and create a rapport to build a foundation for future interactions. When the patient is ambivalent, the goals are to help the patient explore his or her ambivalence, elicit change talk, develop discrepancy, and encourage discussion of future steps. Finally, when the patient is ready, the goals are to strengthen the commitment, elicit change talk, advise and encourage, and negotiation of a plan for action (Roberts, 2005).

"Resistance and change talk are like traffic signals that tell you to go ahead, proceed with caution, slow down, or stop what you are doing" (Miller & Rollnick, 2002) (Figure 4-2). The provider has the capability of assisting the patient along the continuum from not being ready, to being ambivalent, to a level of readiness. The key is to help patients explore where they are and where they want to go, or possibly where they know they do not want to go. The following is an example of the commitment ruler and how it can be used during an encounter:

> Nurse: "I see you are here today to discuss your asthma management. Do you have any concerns you would like to focus on?"
>
> Patient: "Not really. I have had asthma for years and feel pretty comfortable managing it. It just gets away from me sometimes and I have a hard time keeping it under control."
>
> Nurse: "You struggle with keeping your asthma symptoms from worsening at times."
>
> Patient: "That is true. I am good about taking my maintenance medications and always have my rescue inhalers available. I just have a hard time avoiding some of my asthma triggers."
>
> Nurse: "You know what triggers the asthma to worsen, but find it difficult to always avoid them."
>
> Patient: "Well, some triggers are harder than others to avoid. The one I have struggled with for years is my smoking. I just can't seem to kick the habit."
>
> Nurse: "You know it has a negative effect on your breathing, but it is a habit that is difficult to overcome."
>
> Patient: "Exactly."
>
> Nurse: "On a scale of 0 to 10, with 0 being not at all and 10 being most likely, how ready are you to commit to quitting smoking?"
>
> Patient: "I would put myself at a level 7."
>
> Nurse: "I'm curious why you chose a level 7."

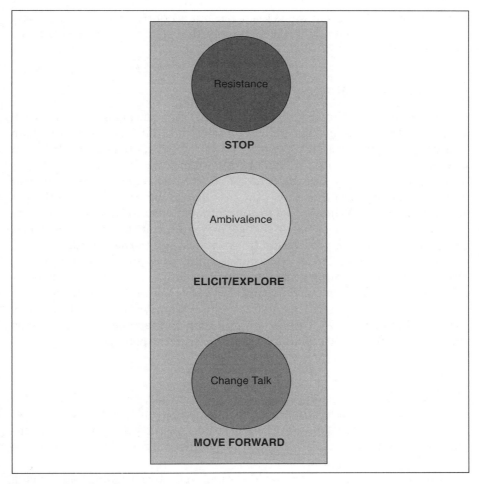

Figure 4-2 Motivational Interviewing Traffic Light

Patient: "Well, I know it's something I need to do for my health, but it's a hard habit to break and I don't feel bad, most of the time. I think if I felt worse, I would have a stronger desire to change."

Nurse: "You clearly have some motivation because you did not put yourself at a level 3, for example. I wonder what it would take for you to get to a level 8 or 9?"

In this example the patient wants to change but is not ready to follow through. Inquiring about what it might take to move further up the scale can promote patient self-exploration.

Communication Skills

Communication is ultimately what motivational interviewing is all about. When proper communication skills are used, a powerful transformation can occur. Granted, motivational interviewing is not just about motivating for behavior change. At times, patients are content with not making changes and are happy with the status quo. In these cases the provider's role is to support the patient and elicit information that allows the provider to better understand the patient's perspectives. When we fail to communicate effectively, we may miss opportunities to promote behavior change, may contribute to patient resistance, and may interfere with progression from ambivalence to change talk.

Motivational interviewing incorporates numerous communication tactics that are vital to promoting behavior change. Failure to use these tools may result in an unsuccessful interaction and fail to assist the patient in evolving. OARS is a mnemonic for Open-ended questions, Affirmation, Reflection, and Summary (Miller & Rollnick, 2002). These communication tools are the basis from which the provider builds a therapeutic relationship with the patient.

OARS

Open-ended questions were previously discussed in Chapter 2. To reiterate, open-ended questions are meant to provoke more detailed answers than a yes or no response. The goal is for the patient to do a majority of the talking. Open-ended questions are a great way to get the conversation started and to keep it going when we meet a dead end.

Affirmation can be demonstrated through reflective listening and through direct statements. This can be as simple as thanking patients for taking the time to talk or for sharing their story. Recognizing that the patient has challenges and his or her management efforts are difficult can reinforce the patient's abilities. Some examples of statements follow:

- "You have a lot on your plate, yet you keep pushing on."
- "You have worked very hard to accomplish your goals."
- "You have a strong spirit and have obviously not let many things get in the way of accomplishing your goals."
- "Your struggles have not been without rewards. You clearly have a drive to reach your goals despite how challenging it may be."

Everyone needs positive feedback for their efforts. Affirmations clarify patient strengths, the motivation that has carried them to this point, and verifies that the provider recognizes the patient's values. Positive reinforcement can evoke self confidence in the patient, which can propel them further in attaining their goals or give them the key that unlocks the desire to change.

Reflection statements are therapeutic but are sometimes difficult to incorporate into a conversation. There are three forms of reflection: simple, amplified, and double-sided. Tone of voice can change the effect of these statements. Be sure not to make the statement sound as if it is a question. Reflections should evoke a sense of understanding, but if the reflection sounds as if it is a question, it cannot be used as it is intended. It is also important to understate an emotion during reflection rather than overstate it:

> Patient: "I know I have hurt my loved ones with my behaviors. It is hard for them to trust me anymore."
> Nurse: "It is difficult when we feel isolated and not have the support of family."
> Patient: "Well, I wouldn't say they aren't supportive because they are. I just feel like they aren't sure I can follow through with this."

A simple reflection is just that. The provider restates what the patient says, showing the patient that he or she is being heard. An amplified reflection is similar to a simple reflection, but the provider "amplifies" or exaggerates what has been said by the patient. This form of reflection may cause the patient to disagree but then go on to further clarify what they meant. The double-sided reflection is more complicated. The provider presents the patient with a reflection on a resistant statement and an earlier statement made by the patient that demonstrated a contradictory statement. Often, patients make statements that are later contradictory and the provider uses this reflection to help the patient see the variable thoughts they have shared.

There are various points in a conversation when it is beneficial to take a moment to summarize what has been stated. At the end of a conversation a summary is provided as part of the conclusion. There are also times of transition during the conversation that may be highlighted by the use of a summary. Summarizing is not only a clear indication that the provider is listening, but also that he or she understands what has been said.

Shifting focus is a tactic that can help ward off resistance. When resistance is detected, the provider can shift topics to focus on a less confrontational topic. The provider is actually more helpful to the patient if the provider avoids topics that trigger resistance.

Rolling with resistance is a common phrase in motivational interviewing. Although it is human nature to become defensive or resist back, it is more therapeutic to just roll with it. Allow the patient to resist. Some patients are highly oppositional at the very start of the encounter. When this occurs it is sometimes more beneficial to verbalize acceptance of the resistance, leading the patient to relax and be less oppositional from that point on.

Reframing is another tactic that can be useful at various points in a conversation. The provider can "invite clients to examine their perceptions in a new light or a reorganized form" (Wagner, & Conners, 2003a). The provider helps the patient to see what he or she is saying in a different light. An example of reframing follows:

> Patient: "I have been trying to take care of things on my own, but my daughter wants to do it all for me. It is driving me crazy, but I don't want to hurt her feelings."
>
> Nurse: "You are trying to manage your disease as independently as possible, but your daughter will not give you the space to do that. Your daughter must love you very much. She cares enough to want to help."
>
> Patient: "Yes, she does love me. I didn't think of it that way."

Another communication tactic is "continuing the paragraph." With effective listening we can hear what the patient is saying, and at times it may be appropriate for the provider to continue the patient's thought. This can contribute to the forward movement of the encounter and promote further exploration of the patient's thoughts about the topic (Roberts, 2005).

Metaphors can be difficult to use appropriately in the course of a conversation, but their use is often helpful to create a picture in the patient's mind to help get a new perspective (Roberts, 2005). The following is an example of how this tool might be used:

> Patient: "I just don't feel like I fit in anymore. I feel very uncomfortable."
>
> Nurse: "It's like being a fish out of water."
>
> Patient: "Yes, I guess you could say that."

There are times in a conversation that it may be important to emphasize the patient's personal choice. Motivational interviewing is patient centered, and to focus on the patient's personal choices, beliefs and values are essential. When the patient is ambivalent, the provider may choose to highlight that personal choice is just as important, if not more important, than facts and figures.

Another communication technique is to side with the negative. When the provider uses this technique the patient may see the faulty thinking and take another look at the positives:

> Patient: "I am not sure I want to quit smoking."
>
> Nurse: "You enjoy it."

Patient: "Well, I'm not sure I would say I enjoy it, but it gives me comfort."

Nurse: "So, what you are saying is that you don't enjoy smoking, but at the same time you are not sure you are ready to give it up because of the comfort it provides you."

Patient: "It doesn't make sense. I don't enjoy it and it's not healthy. And I'm not even sure I would say it is comforting enough to take the risk of continuing."

With so many different communication techniques, the provider is armed with effective tools to evoke behavior change in the patient who is most resistant. Table 4-1 gives examples of those techniques covered in this chapter.

Table 4-1. Communication Techniques

Patient: "I don't know what to think anymore. I tried to do the physical therapy, but the pain was too much to handle. I don't like how the pain medications make me feel. I just don't have a lot of options for managing the pain."

Nurse:

Overstate vs. understate	"You are very frustrated."
Simple reflection	"You are not sure what to think. You have tried the physical therapy and you don't like the medication. You don't feel you have many options to make you feel better."
Amplified reflection	"You are feeling hopeless because of your pain. You are frustrated that the exercise and medication are not good options for you."
Double-sided reflection	"You want to feel better, but it is difficult to do the exercise and medication is not an option for you."
Shifting focus	"You are challenged by your pain. I'm curious what you have done in the past to help you deal with challenges."
Rolling with resistance	"Many people do not like how pain medication makes them feel."
Reframing	"You are frustrated right now, but that is what motivates you to find other ways to manage your pain."
Continuing paragraph	"There may not be a lot of options, but there are some others worth exploring."
Metaphor	"It is like coming to a fork in the road and each option has a roadblock."
Emphasize personal choice	"Medication is not for everyone."
Side with the negative	"Physical therapy is not going to help when you are in too much pain to participate."

SUMMARY

Motivational interviewing is a unique form of interaction that is not without challenges. Understanding the possible traps and barriers assists the provider in being prepared to face these challenges. Also, communication techniques promote effective therapeutic encounters that benefit the patient in his or her journey toward change.

REFERENCES

Botelho, R. (2004). *Motivational practice: Promoting healthy habits and self-care of chronic diseases.* Rochester, NY: MHH Publications.

Levensky, E., Forcehimes, A., O'Donahue, W., & Beitz, K. (2007). Motivational interviewing: An evidence-based approach to counseling helps patients follow treatment recommendations. *American Journal of Nursing, 107*(10), 50–58.

Miller, B. (2004). Values and motivational interviewing: A symposium. *MINUET, 11*(3), 19–20.

Miller, W., & Rollnick, S. (2002). *Motivational interviewing: Preparing people for change* (2nd ed.). New York: The Guilford Press.

Roberts, S. (2005). *Communication for health action: Motivating change* (3rd ed.). Permanente Medical Group.

Rollnick, S., Mason, P., & Butler, C. (1999). *Health behavior change: A guide for practitioners.* Edinburgh: Churchill Livingstone.

Rollnick, S., Miller, W., & Butler, C. (2008). *Motivational interviewing in healthcare: Helping patients change behavior.* New York: The Guilford Press.

Wagner, C., & Conners, W. (2003a). Interaction techniques. Motivational interviewing: Resources for clinicians, researchers, and trainers. Retrieved September 25, 2008, from http://motivationalinterview.org/clinical/interaction.html

Wagner, C., & Conners, W. (2003b). Some mi "traps". Motivational interviewing: Resources for clinicians, researchers, and trainers. Retrieved September 25, 2008, from http://motivationalinterview.org/clinical/traps.html

Zerler, H. (2005). Appreciating confrontation. *MINUET, 12*(2), 18–20.

CHAPTER 5

Developmental Considerations

--- OBJECTIVES ---

After completing this chapter, the reader will be able to

1. Identify the level of Maslow's hierarchy where motivational interviewing tools may be beneficial.
2. Recognize the role of the parent in motivational interviewing, according to the cognitive stage of development.
3. Discuss the role of family on behavior.
4. Determine which stage of parenting behaviors will most likely benefit from the provider working with the parent toward behavior change.
5. Explain how operant conditioning can be used in motivational interviewing.
6. Describe how temperament and parenting affect a child's level of motivation.
7. Identify at least one tactic for the nurse to consider for each stage of development.

--- KEY TERMS ---

Concrete operations
Family systems theory
Formal operations
Human needs theory
Operant conditioning
Personal fable

Preoperational
Reminiscing
Self-actualization
Sensorimotor stage
Temperament

REVIEW OF HUMAN NEEDS THEORY

It is important to understand what drives us to certain behaviors or actions. "Abraham Maslow described human behavior as being motivated by needs that are ordered in a hierarchy" (Polan & Taylor, 2003, p. 69). This theory is not new to nursing and, because of the scope of this text, is only briefly reviewed. The levels of the hierarchy (Polan & Taylor, 2003), beginning with the first level that must be accomplished, are as follows:

- Physiological needs: food, water, shelter
- Safety and security: physical safety, comfort
- Love and belonging: interpersonal relationships
- Self-esteem and the esteem of others: respect, personal achievements
- Self-actualization: highest level of self-esteem, reaching potential

Our goal is to help people to reach that level of **self-actualization**, their highest level of potential. Too often we do not realize our own potential or what we are capable of accomplishing. Our patients are typically stuck somewhere down the ladder. Finding where they are and helping them to discover where they want to go and how they want to get there can prove to be very challenging yet rewarding.

Many people never reach the highest level of Maslow's hierarchy. At the lowest level, physiological needs are priority and need to be met before a person can move toward behavior change. Again, with safety and security, these needs must be met before a person can focus on changing behaviors. The level where motivational interviewing tools can begin to benefit the patient is the level of belonging. This particular level is when the patient and nurse can begin to have an interpersonal relationship that can foster the patient's personal growth to reach the level of self-esteem and, possibly, self-actualization.

The hierarchy pertains to every stage of development. Yet, we can only expect the patient to achieve each level on a continuum, depending on his or her particular stage of development. For example, a 5-year-old having a sense of belonging is not the same as a 30-year-old having a sense of belonging. In this chapter we examine how motivational interviewing tools can be used in each stage of development. Research on motivational interviewing tactics specific to developmental stage is limited and requires further investigation.

COGNITIVE DEVELOPMENT

Not only is it important to understand the theory of human development and what we strive for, but we must also examine the cognitive abilities that allow our successful movement through the hierarchy. Jean Piaget, a psychologist, "described four stages of development related to learning to understand and relate logically to the world" (Leifer & Hartston, 2004, p. 56). Behavior change can only occur when a person has the cognitive ability to understand the effects and consequences of the behavior. During the early stages, when the child is not able to comprehend on a cognitive level, the parent has a primary role in behavior change. As the child advances to a higher cognitive level, he or she becomes more involved in the process. It is important to recognize that although the developmental considerations may change, some issues begin in childhood and are maintained through adulthood, such as obesity (Murtagh, Dixey, & Rudolf, 2006).

The **sensorimotor stage**, from birth to 2 years, is where the parent is the primary participant in behavior change. During this stage the child is learning to interact with his or her environment through the senses and "motor reflex" skills (Polan & Taylor, 2003). The provider may focus on parental behavior change to help shape healthy behaviors in the child from the very beginning.

The **preoperational** stage, from 2 to 6 years, is a time when the child is developing language skills, is self-centered, and is not willing to accept other perspectives. Because of the inability to accept other points of view, the children remain less involved in the encounters with the provider and the parents are the focus of behavior change (Leifer & Hartston, 2004; Polan & Taylor, 2003).

It is during the **concrete operational** stage that children can successfully be involved in behavior change. The age group ranges from ages 6 to 12 years. There is an increased ability to understand more than one piece of information, to think logically, and to problem solve. They can begin to actively participate in a conversation about a negative behavior and independently come up with some possible solutions (Leifer & Hartston, 2004; Polan & Taylor, 2003). Parental involvement is still beneficial, if not necessary.

The fourth and final stage of **formal operations** includes the adolescent group from age 12 years and up. This is a time when the child can think abstractly and hypothetically. They have ability to reason and solve problems (Leifer & Hartston, 2004; Polan & Taylor, 2003). Children of this stage and into adulthood can participate in motivational interviewing independently to promote behavior change.

IT STARTS WITH THE FAMILY

A discussion about the levels of development cannot occur without reviewing the role family plays in a person's development. Family can be those connected biologically, formed through marriage or adoption, or a group of people that live together and share responsibility for each other. "Each family is unique in its style and makeup, but usually attachment and commitment are the features that bind people together" (Polan & Taylor, 2003, p. 32). The **family systems theory** is based on the premise that "what happens to one family member affects the entire family" (Leifer & Hartston, 2004, p. 37). If one member is ill, the entire family is impacted in one way or another. For example, a young mother who has to battle breast cancer may be too fatigued to continue caring for her children. The children are then exposed to another caretaker, even if only temporarily. The normal routine is changed, and the children are forced to adjust to different schedules and rules and also to cope with the emotional impact of having a sick parent.

"The relationship between the individual and the environment is reciprocal; that is, a person's self-concept is affected by the environment in which he or she lives. Self-concept is affected by the individual's stage of development as well" (Polan & Taylor, 2003, p. 12). A person's beliefs arise from the home environment and continue to be built by all that we are exposed to. "Our beliefs are the blueprint from which we construct our lives" (Wright & Leahey, 1994, p. 90). When the nurse sits down with an individual patient, he or she is looking at a compilation of beliefs that are shaped from years of influence. Everything we see, hear, and experience shapes who we are and what we believe. That is then shared with all those around us, and we impact our children's beliefs and then their children's beliefs. Understanding where someone comes from and their basic values benefit the nurse when motivating a patient to change even the smallest behavior. "Beliefs and behavior are intricately connected" (Wright & Leahey, 1994, p. 91). When working with a patient to promote behavior change, family involvement is often beneficial, if not necessary depending on the developmental stage.

The level of influence an event or interaction has on one person may be significantly different from the impact it may have on another person. For example, a brother and sister have both been diagnosed with asthma. For one sibling this can be devastating and difficult to accept, leading to denial and poor management. The other sibling may seek out information to manage the disease and strive to obtain the maximum benefit from treatment. There is never room for assumption that the nurse knows how the patient feels about a situation or diagnosis.

STAGES OF PARENTING BEHAVIORS

Erik Erikson "believed that parents grow as their children develop and are influenced by parent–child interactions at each stage" (Leifer & Hartston, 2004, p. 55). Understanding the stage the parent is in helps the nurse to know what tools may be useful during an interaction. According to Erikson, there are five stages of parenting behaviors:

1. Parental image
2. Authority
3. Integrative
4. Independent teen
5. Departure

In the first stage the parent can visualize themselves as a parent. The second stage is one of questioning their parenting abilities as the child becomes more independent. The third stage is a time when the parent has a sense of responsibility to motivate the child who is gaining independence. The fourth stage incorporates a supportive, yet authoritative role to the teenage child. The fifth and final stage is when the parent can interact with the child as an adult during the time the child is preparing for his or her future as an independent person (Leifer & Hartston, 2004). During the third stage the parent feels a sense of responsibility to motivate the child. It is during this stage that the nurse and parent are most successful as a team to motivate the child toward behavior change. "Motivational Interviewing aimed at affecting parent and/or child behaviors related to a variety of clinical health conditions appears to be feasible as a stand-alone intervention, or incorporated as an adjunctive component in more complex interventions" (Suarez & Mullins, 2008, p. 425).

MOTIVATING THE CHILD

Understanding what motivates a child requires a closer look at the child's **temperament** and the parenting the child receives. Although temperament is reflected through the life span, it is evident as early as birth. Here we examine the importance of temperament in motivational interviewing. Temperament is the "how she behaves, as contrasted to why the individual does what she does (motivation), and how well she does it (ability)" (Chess & Thomas, 1986, p. 4).

Temperament

Different dimensions of temperament help to understand the child's personality. The dimensions are activity, rhythmicity, approach/withdrawal, adaptability, intensity, mood, persistence/attention span, distractibility and sensory threshold (Figure 5-1).

Activity addresses the motor function of the child. This includes but is not limited to activity during sleep, play, awake time, and so on. Consider the toddler who may wake and seems to go immediately into action or the older child who comes home from school and flops onto the couch. The activity level is very different. Some children are even active during sleep as described by restless, thrashing sleep or frequent waking in the night. All these aspects can affect how a child interacts with their environment, which ultimately helps shape his or her behaviors (Carey & McDevitt, 1995; Chess & Thomas, 1986).

Rhythmicity refers to the rhythm of one's life or the schedule one follows day to day. This dimension reflects the physiological functions such as the sleep-wake cycle, hunger/eating, and elimination. Interfering with a child's nap time or trying to communicate with a hungry child will be unsuccessful because he or she cannot focus when tired or hungry. Some do not have predictability of

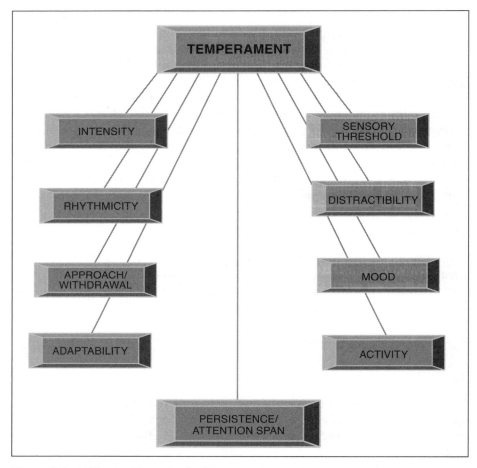

Figure 5-1   Different Dimensions of Temperament

these functions, whereas others need to follow their rhythm and the nurse's role is to ensure the rhythm is not disrupted (Carey & McDevitt, 1995; Chess & Thomas, 1986).

The approach/withdrawal dimension considers how a person responds to a new situation. The approach reactions are positive, and the withdrawal reactions are negative. The child may smile and accept you or may shy away and attempt avoidance. The child may approach new situations wholeheartedly, or the child may require multiple exposures before he or she shows acceptance. This is important to recognize to know when to seek more information or move to another issue or consider offering reinforcement for the current topic (Carey & McDevitt, 1995; Chess & Thomas, 1986).

Adaptability can range from easy to difficult and is a significant character-istic of one's temperament. The child who adapts easily to changes will transi-tion more smoothly. The child who struggles with change will require more support. A child who adjusts to a new situation with little support will likely re-quire less support from the parent and will be more self-motivated. Consider-ation of adaptability can help determine the role the parent will play in behavior change (Carey & McDevitt, 1995; Chess & Thomas, 1986).

Intensity refers to how much stimulation it takes to get a response or how much energy is put into the response. A person described as intense is one who puts an abundance of energy into an action. This is the person who is going to give 100% when working toward a goal. The child may have a meltdown when things do not go as desired or may just move on and focus on something dif-ferent. The child's intensity level can impact how motivated a parent may be to promote behavior change. Parents may want to avoid the intense response they can anticipate when introducing a change in the child's routine (Carey & McDevitt, 1995; Chess & Thomas, 1986).

Mood is variable and can impact one's approach to another person. The child who has a happy, friendly temperament will most likely proceed through an interaction without much difficulty. A negative mood makes it difficult to pro-ceed, and the encounter may need to be rescheduled. Attempting motivational interviewing when a child is exhibiting negative behaviors only leads to frus-tration and failure. Encouraging exploration of a negative mood may be help-ful if the child is capable of understanding how his or her emotions are reflected in his or her actions (Carey & McDevitt, 1995; Chess & Thomas, 1986).

Persistence or attention span can significantly affect the interaction between the nurse and child. Children often have short attention spans. Brief interactions are essential when interacting with the child who has a short attention span. Short, frequent interactions can promote successful exploration of behaviors, motivation, and goal setting. "Persistence refers to the continuation of an activity in the face of obstacles to the maintenance of the activity direction" (Chess & Thomas, 1986, p. 278). The expectation that follow through will occur requires persistence in the child (Carey & McDevitt, 1995; Chess & Thomas, 1986).

Distractibility is another dimension of temperament that is important to consider. When external stimulus interferes with the ability to stay involved in the interaction, the child is distracted. We often attempt to distract from nega-tive behaviors. Providing distraction may be a positive tool for those who are eas-ily distracted but will fail with those who are not easily distracted (Carey & McDevitt, 1995; Chess & Thomas, 1986).

Sensory threshold is "the intensity level of stimulation that is necessary to evoke a discernible response, irrespective of the specific form that the response may take, or the sensory modality affected" (Chess & Thomas, 1986, p. 275). Identifying what it takes to evoke a response from the child helps to determine what possible solutions may be offered to promote behavior change. The parent can help identify productive sources of stimulation to promote action toward positive behaviors (Carey & McDevitt, 1995; Chess & Thomas, 1986).

The previous dimensions of temperament have been considered when developing a construct of the three "clusters" that depict a child's personality. These three types of child are the "difficult" child, the "easy" child, or the "shy" child. Anyone who does not fall into one of these categories is referred to as "intermediate" and encompasses a combination of these characteristics (Carey & McDevitt, 1995; Chess & Thomas, 1986).

The "difficult" child is one who is irregular, intense, negative mood, and slow to adapt or may withdraw from a situation. The "easy" child is easily adaptable, positive mood, and adapts easily to new situations. The "shy" child is also referred to as the "slow to warm up" child and may require additional time to build a therapeutic relationship. An "intermediate" child can have any variety of temperament dimensions that provide the framework of their personality (Carey & McDevitt, 1995; Chess & Thomas, 1986).

The effect of temperament on motivational interviewing has not been thoroughly explored. Research studies are needed to help determine what motivational interviewing tools are best used for the different temperaments to promote the most effective encounter.

Parental Role

Children are clean slates and learn their behaviors from their parents and their environment. "Discipline must have as its basic purpose, the guiding, teaching, or correcting of behavior, not punishment" (Leifer & Hartston, 2004, p. 114). Although parents are disciplining their children, they are essentially promoting behavior change in the home. The parents can be the nurse's ally in promoting behavior change in a child because they have insight into what is effective and what has proven to be ineffective in the home environment.

Tools that are effective in the home environment may be useful for the nurse when promoting behavior change. On the other side, the nurse may be influential in what tools may be transferred to the home environment. When given the option, the child may not desire parent or guardian involvement in the motivational interviewing encounter (Murtagh et al., 2006). The operant theory incorporates the use of positive reinforcement, negative reinforcement, and negative punishment to support effective discipline. "**Operant conditioning**, as described by Skinner, occurs when the learner repeats behaviors that result in a positive outcome of his or her goals and stops behaviors that have negative outcomes" (Leifer & Hartston, 2004, p. 115).

Motivational interviewing incorporates the positive reinforcement of behavior. Offering praise for positive behaviors promotes an internal motivation to receive more praise. When a child receives negative reinforcements, it ultimately promotes more negative behaviors. Children strive for attention, and if most of the attention is on bad behavior, then bad behavior is what the child will most often exhibit. The opportunities to shape a child's behavior are endless. A nurse may have an opportunity to work with children toward changing a number of behaviors, such as hand-washing, nutrition, exercise, or simply any behavior that may promote a healthy lifestyle.

Parents often need support in promoting behavior change. When caring for a child, the nurse must always include the parents. The parents need to continue with the process of behavior change in the home. This requires the parent and nurse to be in agreement about what the problem is, what steps can be realistically taken consistently, and provide feedback on what is effective and what is not effective. In every encounter there should be a "corelationship" between the nurse and patient/family. When the patient is a child, the parent is needed for support of the child and must also evaluate his or her own motivation for changing the child's behavior and how he or she may be influencing the negative behaviors. We cannot expect a child to have healthy behaviors when he or she is not exposed to healthy behaviors at home.

Childhood

Childhood is the time for development of behaviors and a perfect time to focus on promoting healthy behaviors. "The factors impacting patient behavioral outcomes, although complex in adult patients, become even more complicated and multifaceted when addressing pediatric populations" (Suarez & Mullins, 2008, p. 417). The early part of childhood, infancy, toddler, and preschool years is a period of learning, and the parent will be the focus of behavior change. Children in these early stages are not developmentally ready to take on the responsibility to make changes.

School-Aged Child

Childhood considerations are significant for ages 6–12 years. Curiosity is the driving force for this age group. They seek out information and begin making decisions. "The development of moral reasoning happens as the child learns to understand rules and determine if an action is right or wrong" (Leifer & Hartston, 2004, p. 129). Understanding the impact an action can have will help with decision making. The following are some tips to consider when using motivational interviewing with school-aged children:

- Assess the ability to comprehend consequences
- Foster curiosity
- Use more simple reflections than complex reflections

- Assist in forming simple, short-term goals
- Include parents

Assessment is important to ascertain what the child is capable of understanding to help shape the interaction accordingly. If the child does not fully understand an action and how it can affect him or her, it may be important to ask permission to share the necessary information. Reinforcement of the information for the parent to follow through with at home is also necessary. Complete understanding promotes successful goal setting and accomplishment.

Making use of a child's curiosity fosters a rapport between the nurse and child. This shows an interest in what the child finds important. There are times when the nurse has a goal for the encounter and the patient has another agenda. This problem can occur at any developmental stage. Taking the time to focus on the patient's/child's issue provides the time to build a relationship. The child may have a temperament that is "slow to warm up" and the time taken to build that relationship is well spent and will be rewarded in the end with a therapeutic relationship.

Children during this stage of development may not fully understand metaphors. Using simple reflections are best for this age group so that the child can be actively involved in the encounter. Speaking at a level that is not understood will be detrimental because the child may feel uncomfortable asking for an explanation when the nurse is talking to him as if he should understand. Metaphors and complex reflections should be used with caution when interacting with children.

Simple, straightforward goals are best in any stage of development. Children, in particular, need to keep it simple. When children can work toward a simple goal, take steps that are reasonable, and see results in a short period of time, they feel successful. Despite the fact that school-aged children have longer attention spans, they still do not necessarily have more patience to wait for results. The nurse's role is to help the child see even the small rewards with each action.

The parental role in behavior change is extremely important yet variable according to the developmental stage of the child. At this school age the child actually goes through changes from the beginning to the end of this stage in regards to his or her ability to understand rules, make decisions, and develop one's own rules. The parental role ranges from that of making and enforcing rules to that of supporting decisions of what rules to follow and what rules the child may formulate independently. Assessment of the parenting stage is essential to determine the direction the encounter will flow.

MOTIVATING THE ADOLESCENT

Adolescence is a time of discovery, struggles with identity, and gaining independence. This is a time when the nurse can focus more on the patient than the parents as the primary source of change. Motivational interviewing tactics are in many ways the same as with adults. Anticipation of resistance is crucial as the adolescent struggles with independent choices and decision making. Fundamental to this stage of development is the ability to believe they are more powerful than they truly are or have abilities beyond reality. "They may try to manipulate rules, engage in risky behaviors, or deny their own mortality" (Leifer & Hartston, 2004, p.153). It can be challenging to promote behavior change when the patient does not recognize realistic outcomes of negative behaviors (Leifer & Hartston, 2004; Polan & Taylor, 2003).

As with the school-aged child, temperament is important, as is the role of the parent. The parent remains vital to providing rules, but the adolescent is more likely to resist those rules and regulations. The temperament of the parent and the adolescent impact the relationship and determines whether or not there is harmony. "As in music, harmony means many notes that form a pleasant and meaningful relationship" (Chess & Thomas, 1986, p. 97). This relationship helps to determine the level of involvement the parent has when working with the adolescent. When the relationship is tumultuous, the parent may have a negative effect on promoting behavior change. A harmonious relationship between the parent and adolescent often supports parental involvement, with the focus being primarily on the adolescent.

Tips to consider when using motivational interviewing with adolescents are as follows:

- Appreciate resistance
- Recognize ambivalence
- Encourage independence
- Discourage unrealistic thinking
- Use more simple reflections than complex reflections
- Offer positive reinforcement

Adolescents tend to resist being part of a family and holding the family beliefs in entirety. They search to become individuals and strive to formulate their own beliefs. It is vital to embrace the resistance or "roll with resistance" when working directly with adolescents. Seek to understand who they are and what makes them unique as individuals. During a time when they are struggling with what beliefs they want to incorporate into their self-concept, the nurse must be nonjudgmental and foster an environment where the adolescent feels comfortable and confident in expressing his or her ideas (Leifer & Hartston, 2004; Polan & Taylor, 2003).

Ambivalence is a hallmark of adolescence. It is a time when there is movement away from the family, yet they continue to need love, support, and guidance from their parents (Polan & Taylor, 2003). Recognizing ambivalence as it is related to the developmental stage is helpful to understand when the adolescent is struggling with making choices. Exploring this ambivalence may be necessary to move forward toward discovery of ambivalence about a particular issue.

Independence is a goal of the adolescent stage. The nurse should encourage movement toward independence in determining what behaviors the adolescent may want to keep, modify, or avoid altogether. When the adolescent perceives the nurse is respecting his or her perspectives and fostering his or her independence, a strong alliance can be formed. The nurse and adolescent can then move toward behavior change (Leifer & Hartston, 2004; Polan & Taylor, 2003).

Often, the adolescent has unrealistic goals because he or she feels invincible. Adolescents recognize that others can be harmed by risky behaviors but believe they are immune to the negative consequences. This is referred to as the "**personal fable.**" Discouraging goal setting based on this false sense of immunity promotes a more successful outcome. Caution must be taken when trying to avoid feeding into this belief to maintain a therapeutic relationship (Bastable, 2006).

Adolescents can think more abstractly and comprehend more complex concepts. They can understand more than just simple reflections. It is important to incorporate some of the more complex reflections and metaphors and not use only the simple reflections. By using more complex reflections, it helps adolescents to explore issues at different levels and begin to use these more advanced thought processes to formulate their personal goals and steps toward goal achievement (Leifer & Hartston, 2004; Polan & Taylor, 2003).

Positive reinforcement has a place in every motivational interviewing interaction. The adolescent, in particular, strives to achieve a positive response from parents and peers. The peer response takes priority for the adolescent. The nurse can take advantage of this characteristic and focus on the positive actions the adolescent takes to achieve acceptance of his or her peers. The adolescent may present multiple behaviors that represent a compilation of behaviors shared with his or her peers. Focusing on those positive behaviors and giving praise helps to build the adolescent's self-confidence and, hopefully, achieve positive outcomes.

MOTIVATING THE ADULT

Just as in childhood, there are different stages of adulthood. What drives adults vary depending on their stage of development. The younger adult will have different goals and motivating factors than that of an older adult. Younger adults are often at a point where they seek out information to promote healthy lifestyles or may be still taking risks that could negatively affect their health. The older adult may be more focused on chronic illness and attempting to prevent long-term complications. Awareness of these differences will prove to be helpful when promoting behavior change through motivational interviewing. Finding a common ground between the priorities of the chronic illness, personal priorities, and implementing changes can be challenging (Bastable, 2006; O'Connor, Stacey, & Legare, 2008).

"As in the child or adolescent, temperament in the adult is a significant factor in shaping the person's style of coping with the daily routines of living" (Chess & Thomas, 1986, p. 101). Temperament, alone, is not responsible for one's personality or behavior issues. It is "the consonance or dissonance between the person's characteristics, abilities, and motivations and the expectations and demands of the environment" (Chess & Thomas, 1986, p. 103). Consider the patient with the low activity level who is obese and coping with type 2 diabetes and struggling with the idea of incorporating exercise into his or her daily routine. This person will likely be resistant to the nurse encouraging exercise. Motivational interviewing skills are essential in this situation.

The adult, as an independent decision maker, has the primary role in the motivational interviewing encounter. The basic tactics of motivational interviewing can be used throughout adulthood. The family plays an essential role in supporting actions toward healthy behavior but is not the focus of the interaction. Adult and adolescent patients benefit from all motivational interviewing strategies.

Young Adulthood

The young adult is between 20 and 40 years old. Important aspects of this developmental stage is that young adults are often beginning to support themselves and live independently, possibly starting a family, and building careers. Interactions with young adults may focus on disease prevention, role transitions, disease management, or issues related to the stressors of managing a home, family, career, and possibly chronic illness (Bastable, 2006; Leifer & Hartston, 2004; Polan & Taylor, 2003). The topics of interest are endless. Some special considerations for this stage of development are as follows:

- Assess where the young adult is in regards to school, work, relationships, and level of independence to help determine at what level of Maslow's hierarchy the patient resides.
- Foster self-reflection
- Recognize ambivalence.
- Encourage family support.
- Use more complex reflections than simple reflections.
- Offer positive reinforcement.
- Use the importance ruler.

By the time the adolescent enters this stage, he or she has developed a strong self-concept. Those becoming independent will have their basic needs as a priority. The young adult who has begun a family may be more focused on Maslow's stage of safety and security or interpersonal relationships. Some may even be at the point of successfully establishing self-esteem and respect for others. Getting to know the patient and building a rapport are vital. There are so many paths the young adult may be on that there is no room for assumptions (Bastable, 2006; Leifer & Hartston, 2004; Polan & Taylor, 2003).

"The cognitive capacity of young adults is fully developed, but with maturation, they continue to accumulate new knowledge and skills through formal and informal experiences" (Bastable, 2006, p. 126). It is important to support the young adult as he or she analyzes, problem solves, makes independent decisions, and appreciates consequences of health behaviors. This is a period of time that is full of decisions about health, family, and career. The nurse's role is to help the patient through the process of introspection as he or she faces numerous decision-making opportunities. This promotes forward movement toward behaviors that will assist the patient in meeting personal goals.

Ambivalence occurs throughout the life span. This is the driving force of motivational interviewing. During times of ambivalence the nurse can explore the ambivalence and appreciate it as being a natural occurrence. When there is a behavior that is determined to be detrimental by the patient, proper communication techniques assist in exploring the patient's feelings about continuing the behavior versus changing the behavior. Exploring with the patient is always more successful than providing information to make changes the nurse may see as pertinent.

Family support is beneficial, although not necessary, in the young adult stage. Involvement of the family at any stage of development should be encouraged by the nurse. "Nurses can be the catalyst to facilitate communication between family members or between the family and other healthcare professionals" (Wright & Leahey, 1994, p. 109). Whether the young adult is a parent, married with no children, or single, family is affected by the patient's behaviors and vice versa. As stated previously, everyone in the family unit is touched by a person's health issues, risk behaviors, and health-related choices. Recruiting support of the family can only enhance the outcome of an encounter for behavior change.

Motivational interviewing incorporates use of reflections to demonstrate the nurse is listening and understands what the patient has stated. Reflections also help the patient to see a new perspective. More complex reflections can be used at this stage because the young adult is most often capable of fully understanding metaphors and abstract thoughts. Miller and Rollnick (2002) recommend use of more complex reflections to fewer simple reflections. This would certainly be appropriate for any of the adult stages.

Positive reinforcement is essential in all stages of development. Hearing praise for constructive actions promotes continuation of those particular actions and attempts for higher goals. For example, the patient may be overwhelmed by all the stressors in his or her life. The patient has been working hard to attain a personal health goal but has been distracted by all the stressors. The nurse should point out the positive aspects of a situation that may have been overlooked by the patient. This praise can be the pivotal point for the patient to refocus and move forward on the momentum created by the optimistic feelings that are born out of praise.

One study looked at the college-aged student and the utilization of the importance ruler versus readiness to change. Both tools were found to be effective. The importance ruler and confidence ruler used in motivational interviewing is based on the 10-point Likert scale. The results of the study support use of the importance ruler as a valid tool to assess motivation (Harris, Walters, & Leahy, 2008). The participants were young adults and the findings can be used in this age group. Further research is needed to compare these tools in other developmental stages (Harris et al., 2008).

Middle Adulthood

The middle-aged adult is between the ages of 40 and 65 years. The goals during this stage of development typically are different from those of young adulthood. The exceptions to this rule are the older woman who is either adding to her family or even, possibly, beginning her family. Often, the career is established, as well as a strong sense of self. The children are typically older and may be in or out of the home. For those whose children are out of the home, there may be new interests and further self-exploration and reflection on the past, present, and future goals (Bastable, 2006; Leifer & Hartston, 2004; Polan & Taylor, 2003).

Special considerations for motivational interviewing with the middle-aged adult are as follows:

- Foster a therapeutic relationship for the patient to openly re-examine their personal goals
- Encourage exploration of the past
- Explore ambivalence
- Anticipate resistance
- Use more complex reflections than simple reflections
- Encourage a sense of accomplishment

The middle-aged adult is at the stage of development where the past can be reviewed and a future outlook can help to re-create behavior goals. The nurse needs to foster a therapeutic relationship in which the patient feels comfortable in evaluating current or future goals. Being nonjudgmental and respectful of the patient's personal beliefs and objectives foster such a relationship. The road we have traveled often points us in the direction we will follow for future travels.

The nurse should recognize that there is history of successful and failed attempts at behavior change. These experiences help shape patients' self-esteem and ultimately impact what they believe they can accomplish when setting new goals. Encouraging patients to explore their past is of the essence. Knowing what has worked well in the past promotes successful goal setting and attainment. Being aware of the actions that were unsuccessful allows the patient to avoid those actions in the future. Avoiding past failures does not guarantee future success but helps to keep from repeating mistakes and allows patients to further explore their possibilities for success. Another important factor with this developmental stage is the risk of "midlife crisis" when the patient may engage in atypical behaviors in an attempt to make up for missed opportunities. These behaviors are likely to promote a false sense of well-being, and the nurse must be careful not to alienate the patient who has altered viewpoints related to this crisis phase (Leifer & Hartston, 2004).

Having the past history of successes and failures provides the patient with more ammunition to be ambivalent. They have seen more benefits and negative consequences. This gives the patient more to contemplate and weigh when determining what may require change and what steps may be successful. There are always pros and cons to making a lifestyle change. The patient may be ambivalent due to negative experiences, lack of knowledge, lack of foresight of the positive effects of the behavior change, and personal fears. Understanding the cause of the middle-aged adult's ambivalence can help the nurse to know where to guide the encounter.

Resistance is inevitable at any stage of development. Resistance at this stage is common. The middle-aged adult has witnessed negative aspects of a behavior, may lack insight of the potential positive outcomes, or may lack the support system to help carry them through the difficult phases of behavior change. Recognizing and embracing the resistance encourages the patient to fully explore why he or she is resistant and potentially move forward to search for experiences that may be more positive and lead to more victorious outcomes.

Complex reflections should be used more often than simple reflections with the middle-aged adult, as well as the young adult. Simple reflections at this stage of development can provide the sense of understanding from the nurse that is necessary to build rapport. The more complex reflections bring out a deeper thought process in patients as they explore what they are capable of accomplishing (Miller & Rollnick, 2002).

During the middle-aged adult stage of development, patients examine where they have been and what they have accomplished. "Middle-aged adults, in fact, may choose to modify aspects of their lives that they perceive as unsatisfactory or adopt a new lifestyle as a solution to dissatisfaction" (Bastable, 2006, p. 129). This is an opportunity for the nurse to encourage that sense of accomplishment. When people feel good about where they have been, they are more likely to believe they have an ability to go further and accomplish whatever goals they set before them. The nurse can offer praise for the accomplishments, help the patient to determine what made the accomplishments successful, and help the patient transfer those skills and abilities to achieve new goals.

Older Adulthood

The older adult population is 65 years of age and older. "Most older persons suffer from at least one chronic condition, and many have multiple conditions" (Bastable, 2006, p. 130). These chronic conditions, along with changes in self-image due to change in physical characteristics, family roles, and transitions from careers to retirement, all provide opportunities for the nurse to support behavior change. During this time the patient may feel despair due to the inability to reach previous goals or a sense of accomplishment for all that the patient has done over his or her lifetime. Self-care promotion is vital during this developmental stage. Every day they make decisions and exhibit behaviors that affect their health. During chronic illness it becomes a greater issue to have the skills to be autonomous in self-management and rely more on the health professional for support and fill the knowledge gaps (Kennedy, Rogers, & Bower, 2007).

Special considerations for motivational interviewing in older adulthood are as follows:

- Encourage the patient to reminisce
- Promote active involvement in decision making
- Recognize barriers
- Focus on wellness
- Appreciate the patient's history

The older adult comes to each encounter with a wealth of past experience that has helped to shape his or her current perspectives. "In working with older adults, **reminiscing** is a beneficial approach to use to establish a therapeutic relationship" (Bastable, 2006, p. 135). It is important to encourage older adults to look at their past and draw from their most powerful memories. This may bring about new perspectives toward tackling a goal. The information shared can provide the nurse with numerous tools to help promote behavior change by increasing the understanding of who the patient is and his or her abilities and deepest concerns. Reminiscing can stimulate patients to reassess where they are and what personal goals they will set for themselves (Bastable, 2006).

The nurse should promote active involvement of the older adult in decision making. Often, older adults feel a loss of control because of physical changes that cause them to be less independent, as well as role changes that typically occur. Patients may be forced to be more independent because of their spouse becoming more dependent, or they may be more dependent due to illness or physical disability. Encouraging involvement in decision making increases the patient's self-esteem and improves the self-concept, which provides momentum toward healthy behavior change (Bastable, 2006; Leifer & Hartston, 2004; Polan & Taylor, 2003).

It is important to recognize the numerous barriers that affect the older adult. Financial restraints can have a negative impact on self-care. A patient may not take a prescribed medication because he or she simply cannot afford it. Physical barriers must also be considered. The patient who has limited resources may be more isolated. Isolation often leads to depression, which can significantly affect one's motivation level. Cognitive changes, such as dementia, can also interfere with one's ability to actively participate in behavior change. "Earlier theorists believed disengagement was a task of the older adult" (Leifer & Hartston, 2004, p. 202). Anticipation of this disengagement or isolation of the older adult can help to overcome this particular barrier (Bastable, 2006; Leifer & Hartston, 2004; Polan & Taylor, 2003).

A focus on wellness during the older adult stage is different from a focus on wellness in the young adult. "The emphasis is no longer solely prevention but health maintenance" (Polan & Taylor, 2003, p. 246). As stated previously, the older adult is likely to have at least one chronic disease. Prevention now incorporates long-term complications of such chronic diseases. Older adults are likely to be struggling with ambivalence about disease management and maintaining their current health status and possibly improving their overall health. Wellness encompasses both maintenance and improvement of health (Leifer & Hartston, 2004; Polan & Taylor, 2003).

When working with older adults, the nurse should always appreciate their history. "The teacher (nurse) should recognize the lifelong accomplishments of the older adult, be nonjudgmental, and foster an environment conducive to learning" (Leifer & Hartston, 2004, p. 205). When older adults can feel accomplished, they are in a positive mindset, and this is essential to the success of a motivational interviewing encounter.

SUMMARY

A person's developmental stage is important to take into account when promoting behavior change through the use of motivational interviewing. The developmental stage helps to determine the level of involvement for parents and families to be considered (Figure 5-2). Although some aspects of a person's temperament are sustained through a lifetime, some aspects can evolve over time. Over the course of this text, we examine this consideration of developmental stage through examples in the later chapters.

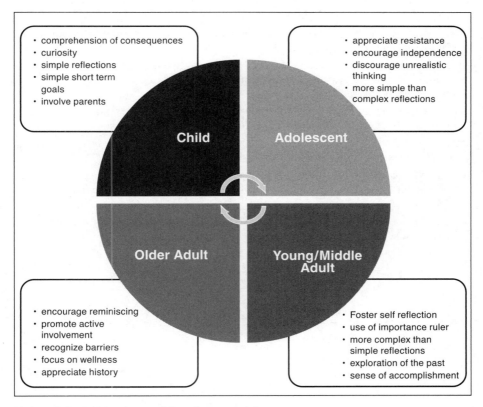

Figure 5-2 Motivation and Developmental Stage

REFERENCES

Bastable, S. (2006). *Essentials of patient education.* Sudbury, MA: Jones and Bartlett.

Carey, W., & McDevitt, S. (1995). *Coping with children's temperament: A guide for professionals.* New York: Basic Books.

Chess, S., & Thomas, A. (1986). *Temperament in clinical practice.* New York: The Guilford Press.

Harris, T. R., Walters, S., & Leahy, M. (2008). Readiness to change among a group of heavy-drinking college students: Correlates of readiness and a comparison of measures. *Journal of American College Health, 57*(3), 325–330.

Kennedy, A., Rogers, A., & Bower, P. (2007). Support for self care for patients with chronic disease. *British Medical Journal, 335*(7627), 968–970.

Leifer, G., & Hartston, H. (2004). Growth and development across the lifespan: A health promotion focus. St. Louis, MO: Saunders.

Miller, W., & Rollnick, S. (2002). *Motivational interviewing: Preparing people for change* (2nd ed.). New York: The Guilford Press.

Murtagh, J., Dixey, R., & Rudolf, M. (2006). A qualitative investigation into the levers and barriers to weight loss in children: Opinions of obese children. *Archives of Disease in Childhood, 91*, 920–923.

O'Connor, A., Stacey, D., & Legare, F. (2008). Coaching to support patients in making decisions. *British Medical Journal, 336*(7638), 228–229.

Polan, E., & Taylor, D. (2003). *Journey across the lifespan: Human development and health promotion.* Philadelphia: F.A. Davis.

Suarez, M., & Mullins, S. (2008). Motivational interviewing and pediatric health behavior interventions. *Journal of Developmental & Behavioral Pediatrics, 29*(5), 417–428.

Wright, L., & Leahey, M. (1994). *Nurses and families: A guide to family assessment and intervention.* Philadelphia: F.A. Davis.

Motivational Interviewing in Cardiac Health

INTRODUCTION

Cardiovascular disease can have devastating effects on a person's life. "An estimated 80,000,000 American adults (one in three) have one or more types of cardiovascular disease" (**American Heart Association**, 2009, p. 6). Given these statistics we can assume that most everyone has been touched by cardiac disease.

Each patient is someone's mother/father, sister/brother, daughter/son, wife/ husband, or friend. "Nearly 2,400 Americans die of CVD [cardiovascular disease] each day, an average of one death every 37 seconds and claims as many lives as cancer, chronic lower respiratory diseases, accidents and diabetes combined" (American Heart Association, 2009, p. 7). Cardiovascular disease, including stroke, is a major cause of death in the United States. It is also one that is highly preventable. Interestingly, if every form of major cardiovascular disease were eliminated, Americans could add another 7 years onto their life expectancy. Clearly, a focus on prevention, maintenance, and treatment is of the utmost importance (American Heart Association, 2009; Centers for Disease Control and Prevention [CDC], 2009).

The U.S. Department of Health and Human Services reports statistics related to **hypertension** and total cholesterol. The prevalence of hypertension increases with age. Between 2003 and 2006, 36% of the population between the ages of 45 and 54 and 65% of men and 80% of women over 75 years of age had hypertension. The percentage of the population with elevated total cholesterol (>240 mg/dL) has decreased over time. Women are more likely to suffer from elevated cholesterol than are men (National Center for Health Statistics, 2009).

Cardiovascular disease is very costly, and in our present economy it is vital to maintain costs. Increasing healthy behaviors and decreasing the incidence of cardiovascular disease will help decrease our country's medical costs. Costs projected for 2009 for cardiovascular disease and stroke are greater than $475 billion. These costs include healthcare costs and costs of decreased productivity, whether by death or disability. Controlling healthcare costs and improving the health of our nation are among our priorities (American Heart Association, 2009; CDC, 2009).

The previous statistics, among others, have put heart disease and stroke on the list of the focus areas for Healthy People 2010. Healthy People 2010's leading health indicators such as physical activity and obesity help guide our practice. "CDC's work is grounded in goals and strategies set forth in Healthy People 2010, the Division for Heart Disease and Stroke Prevention's strategic plan, and the landmark publication *A Public Health Action Plan to Prevent Heart Disease and Stroke*" (CDC, 2009). Data available through **DATA2010** (the database for Healthy People 2010) was produced from initiatives set forth by Healthy People 2010 and are directly related to heart disease. This data can help point us in the right direction to improve our country's cardiac health. Data collected up to this point are from 2005. More data need to be collected and documented before criteria for Healthy People 2020 can be developed. The data include, but are not limited to, information regarding blood cholesterol screening, heart failure-related hospitalizations, and health behavior counseling to include physical activity, smoking cessation, and healthy nutrition (CDC, 2009; see also www.healthypeople.gov/About/hpfact.htm).

According to the CDC, the average blood cholesterol level is 202 mg/dL. "A ten percent decrease in total cholesterol levels (population wide) may result in an estimated thirty percent reduction in the incidence of CHD (**coronary heart disease**)" (CDC, 2009). Ninety percent of persons know whether they have high blood pressure, and 93% are taking action to control their blood pressure. Data also tell us that "about 69% of people who have a first heart attack, 77% who have their first stroke and 74% with congestive heart failure have blood pressure higher than 140/90 mm Hg" (American Heart Association, 2009, p. 18). These data highlight the need to focus on improving the population's cardiovascular health. Promoting individual behavior change through motivational interviewing will improve the overall statistics and enhance the health of our nation.

CHALLENGES IN CARDIOVASCULAR DISEASE

There are many challenges to managing and preventing cardiovascular disease as well as numerous barriers to achieving cardiovascular health (Figure 6-1). One important factor is that the signs and symptoms are often silent. The patient does not necessarily feel bad, yet he or she may be at risk for death or disability caused by cardiac disease or stroke. We need something to motivate us, and these motivating factors are often physical symptoms. When we do not feel well, we take

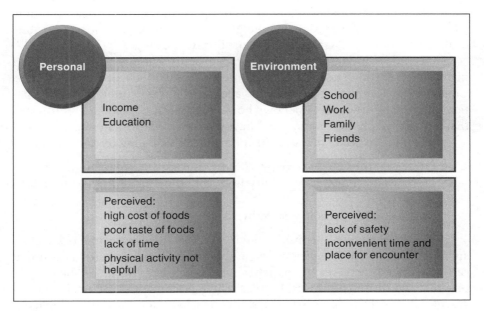

Figure 6-1 Barriers to Cardiovascular Health

Source: Adapted from: Gatewood, J., et. al., 2008.

action to feel better. When we feel good, we do not have the physical reminders of the need to improve our cardiac health. "Behavioral changes that prevent or minimize signs and symptoms and disease progression are just as important as the medications prescribed to treat the heart failure and the most difficult lifestyle changes include smoking cessation, weight loss, and restriction of dietary sodium" (Paul & Sneed, 2004, p. 305).

Too often, the symptoms that may alert us to a problem are not obvious, or we do not realize their connection to cardiac health. Cardiac disease can be independent of other factors or may come as a complication of other diseases, such as diabetes. This can complicate matters for the patient because of the overwhelming effect it can have when trying to manage multiple chronic diseases. Cardiovascular problems include heart failure, **congenital heart disease**, stroke, **peripheral vascular disease**, **peripheral arterial disease**, hypertension, and dyslipidemia. When patients do not follow treatment recommendations, the cardiac disease can worsen: This is the most frequent reason for rehospitalization. Motivational interviewing has been found to be effective in assessing a patient's readiness to change and subsequently moving toward change at an appropriate time for the individual (Paul & Sneed, 2004).

As with any issue that requires behavior change, the perceived risk must outweigh the benefits of staying in their present lifestyle. Lack of physical energy or other health problems may make it difficult to put forth the time and effort toward a patient's self-management of his or her cardiovascular disease. Finding what drives each patient to make changes or maintain status quo can be quite challenging, but it is essential to promote behavior change.

Time and location of treatment is often a factor that interferes with patient involvement in care. There should be some variability in scheduling encounters. Consider the telephone encounter that allows the nurse to interact with the patient in the comfort of his or her own home. Kreman et al. (2006) demonstrated that a single telephone session could have a positive effect on lipid profiles and activity level. This study revealed the following encouraging outcomes:

- Decreased total cholesterol by 37.5 mg/dL, or a 15% reduction
- Decreased average low-density lipoprotein by 28.33 mg/dL, or a 17% reduction
- Physical fitness level increased by 13%

It is also important to consider the risk factors involved. Some risk factors are not modifiable, such as gender, age, and genetics. Focusing on risk factors that can be reduced increases the patient's self-esteem because he or she can see progress and formulate workable goals. The modifiable risk factors in cardiovascular disease include smoking, dyslipidemia, hypertension, physical inactivity, obesity, and diabetes (Gatewood et al., 2008).

When looking to increase compliance on the part of the patient, the American Heart Association (2009) recommends the following motivational interviewing tactics:

- Patient involvement
- Monitor progress at each encounter
- Ask questions that stimulate the conversation
- Create an encounter based on the patient's current age, gender, values/ beliefs, attitudes, and personal situations

These tactics can be very useful when conducting a motivational interview with a patient.

BENEFITS OF SELF-MANAGEMENT

Patients need to have some control over their health and well-being. People tend to feed off previous successes. When they feel dependent on others and lack control over their own health, they are not likely to be motivated to make changes to improve their health. One study looked at patients with chronic heart failure and their limitations in physical activity and independence. Not only do we need to consider the measurable factors when evaluating a person's cardiac status, we need to consider quality of life. The study evaluated the use of motivational interviewing to improve quality of life. The findings were significant for trends toward improving self-efficacy and motivation level to achieve increased physical activity (Brodie, Inoue, & Shaw, 2008).

Another study also evaluated quality of life and self-care in patients with advanced heart failure. The interventions were performed by nurses. The nurses worked with inpatients to provide a supportive educational intervention. Although immediate effect was not noticeable, the self-care behavior in the intervention group was higher at the time of follow-up. This was not a reflection of a change in ability but demonstrated a true behavior change (Jaarsma et al., 2000).

Studies have shown what motivational interviewing can do. Another study evaluated the effects of motivational interviewing in the cardiac rehabilitation patient and also determined whether patients found this to be an acceptable technique. The results are not surprising. The patients participated and often wanted to continue past the allotted 10-minute session. The study personnel stated the "patients just don't stop talking . . . they love the undivided time and attention." This is often the case when motivational interviewing is used. Patients open up and share information about themselves and their disease management that is not seen when the conversation is nurse driven (Everett, Davidson, Sheerin, Salamonson, & DiGiacomo, 2008).

CASE STUDIES

The following case studies capture a brief intervention between the nurse and patient. Note the differences between the two encounters for each case study.

Case Study 1

The patient is newly diagnosed with cardiac disease after suffering a myocardial infarction without precipitating symptoms. Behavior change is often necessary to improve patient health and decrease the risk of another myocardial infarction.

Interaction Without Motivational Interviewing

Nurse: Good morning. How are you doing today?

Patient: I'm lousy. I just want to go home.

Nurse: I can help you with that. We have a few things we need to go over before you are discharged. I'd like to start with reviewing some of your medications and then we can talk about your exercise and nutrition that can help prevent another heart attack.

Patient: Okay.

Nurse: I made you a list of medications and how often you need to take them.

Patient: Why do I need to take all those medications?

Nurse: Your doctor has prescribed them for you and my job is to make sure you understand how and when you need to take them.

Patient: Well, okay.

Nurse: (reads from list of medications and medication schedule) Now we need to talk a little about exercise. Do you get routine exercise?

Patient: Not really. I work so many hours that I don't have the energy for a specific exercise routine.

Nurse: So, you need to find a little time each day to do some exercise. Exercise can be walking, jogging, swimming, aerobics, but I would start with a simple activity such as walking. You should walk for 15 minutes each day and build up to 30 minutes each day. If you can do more, that would be great.

Patient: Okay.

Nurse: Nutrition is also important. You will need to eat a low fat, low cholesterol, high fiber diet. Try to eat lower calories so you can lose weight because that is not good for your heart health.

Patient: Wow, this is a lot to change.

Nurse: That is true, but it is so important to take care of your heart. You don't want to end up here in the hospital again.

Patient: You are right about that.

Motivational Interviewing Interaction

Nurse: Good morning. I thought I would stop in to see how you are feeling and possibly talk about what it is going to take to get you on the road to recovery and discharged home.

Patient: Well, I can't wait to go home. What is it going to take for me to get home?

Nurse: We have a cardiac rehabilitation program that you may find helpful and is recommended by the doctors.

Patient: I don't want to participate in a program. I just want to go home! (Resistance)

Nurse: You have been through a lot these past couple days. You must feel overwhelmed with all the testing and education you are receiving.

Patient: You are right about that!

Nurse: It can be difficult when we long to be home, but we also know it is important to learn about prevention, so this will not happen again.

Patient: Well, I don't want it to happen again, that's for sure, but I don't see how I can prevent it when I don't know what caused it to begin with. This is all very frustrating. (Ambivalence)

Nurse: You feel you don't understand what happened or how you got here and that makes it almost impossible to know how to prevent it from happening again.

Patient: That's just it. I felt fine the day before all this happened. I have been healthy and active all my life. It's almost useless to try to be healthy when something like this can just hit you out of the blue!

Nurse: There's a feeling of hopelessness and helplessness that goes along with having a heart attack, and most patients feel that way. Maybe you can share with me what you have done in the past to deal with feelings of helplessness.

Patient: Hmm. I don't know. Normally, I would get up and do something about the problem, but I just don't have the energy. I don't have any fight in me.

Nurse: Where do you think that fight has gone?

Patient: It left when my heart stopped working. I guess I'm afraid that if I fight this or do anything physical, that my heart is going to stop again, but this time I might not make it.

Nurse: (silence)

Patient: I never thought I could be so afraid of something. I've always been the strong one in my family, and now they will see me as weak and fragile.

Nurse: We all have a fragile side to us. It is normal to have fears. On one hand you are afraid and want to just lie here and let life pass you by, but on the other hand, you feel a sense of responsibility to your family and need to be involved.

Patient: I guess you are right. Maybe you could tell me about the rehab program. (Change talk)

Discussion

The two scenarios for case study 1 are different in many ways. Given the differences in all individuals, these interactions could have a variety of paths to take. The first scenario demonstrates an ineffective encounter for behavior change. The nurse dominates the conversation and directs where the conversation goes. This was clearly not a patient-centered interaction. You can see how the patient became passive with responses of "okay," as if he felt a need to agree with the nurse. The nurse did not promote participation from the patient and did not offer support when the patient was obviously feeling overwhelmed. When the patient brought up concerns about barriers to exercise, the nurse disregarded it and told the patient to figure it out. This patient did not fully understand the medications or why he was taking them. The nurse again disregarded this important factor that should be addressed with all patients. It would have been a perfect opportunity to explore the barriers and help the patient come up with some possible solutions. The patient was not really considered when the nurse set forth the goals for him to achieve. Better listening skills, more supportive statements, and patient involvement would have improved this encounter tremendously.

The second scenario demonstrates how motivational interviewing is respectful of the patient's needs and desires. The nurse recognized the patient's ambivalence and helped to explore it. The patient was more open to suggestions or information when he found the nurse to show interest and care about his thoughts and feelings. There was a good rapport between the patient and nurse. The nurse did not pressure the patient to receive information. She let the patient decide when he was ready to learn more about the cardiac rehabilitation program. The second scenario was a more successful encounter and produced more positive results. Key statements from the patient indicated resistance, ambivalence, or readiness to make a change. Motivational interviewing is not strict in how it is used, and each encounter has the potential to be successful or ineffective. It is important to maintain the basic tactics of motivational interviewing to achieve maximum potential for behavior change.

Case Study 2

The patient had a **stroke** 6 months ago. The physician has made a variety of recommendations for behavior change to improve the patient's mobility and decrease the risk of repeated stroke. The patient has not yet made any changes.

Interaction Without Motivational Interviewing

> Nurse: Good morning. I understand you are here today for us to talk about some changes your doctor has asked you to make. Could you tell me how you are doing with those changes or what difficulties you have had making those changes?
>
> Patient: I can't even remember everything they told me I need to do different. I don't know how they thought I could make so many changes.
>
> Nurse: You do realize how important it is to follow the doctor's recommendations to prevent another stroke, right?
>
> Patient: I know I need to make some changes. I just don't know where to start.
>
> Nurse: Well, I'm going to start by talking with you about your activity level. How much exercise do you get a week?
>
> Patient: I work at a desk for 8 hours a day. I do not get much exercise at all, except on the weekends when I have more time.
>
> Nurse: It is not good to sit for such long periods of time. You really need to get some exercise throughout the day. Why don't you take a walk break every hour?
>
> Patient: That is not always possible. I can't just leave to go for a walk whenever I want to.
>
> Nurse: I would recommend you find a way to get more exercise. Now let's talk about the smoking. When do you plan on quitting?
>
> Patient: I don't know. It's a hard habit to break.
>
> Nurse: I'm sure it is, but it is so important in preventing another stroke from happening.
>
> Patient: That's what you keep telling me.
>
> Nurse: I just want to check with you about your medication. Are you taking it the way the doctor told you to?
>
> Patient: Yes.
>
> Nurse: Good. Keep taking your medication, get some exercise and work hard at quitting smoking. We'll talk more at the next visit.

Motivational Interviewing Interaction

Nurse: Good morning. I'm wondering how you have been feeling and if there is anything I can help you with today.

Patient: Well, I know the doctor wants me to make some changes, but I just haven't had time to deal with it all.

Nurse: It is especially hard to find time to do something we really aren't sure we want to do.

Patient: Oh, I do want to do some things different, but there is just so much that he asked me to do that whenever I think about it, I just get overwhelmed and can't even think about it. And I really can't think about having another stroke. (Ambivalence)

Nurse: (silence)

Patient: I still can't believe I had a stroke.

Nurse: It is hard to get behind something that just doesn't seem real.

Patient: That's true.

Nurse: Could I ask if there is one thing that you could change, what would it be?

Patient: Yes, I think I would be able to use my right arm better. But I can't do those exercises they told me to do. (Resistance)

Nurse: Often, starting out is difficult, and if we can't do it perfect, there seems no reason to put forth the effort.

Patient: I agree that starting out is hard, but it would be worth it if I could improve my arm at all.

Nurse: You want to improve the use of your right arm. You have been given some exercises, but up to this point, you haven't done them routinely.

Patient: That's correct. Maybe I could make a schedule so I can at least try to do them a few times a week. (Change talk)

Nurse: That's a great place to start. I'm confident that once you set your mind to it and get started, that you will accomplish your goal.

Patient: Thank you. I'm actually looking forward to this.

Discussion

The previous two scenarios for case study 2 have some significant differences, and it is obvious that some tactics are not effective. However, the use of motivational interviewing is more successful in promoting behavior change in the patient who has suffered a stroke.

In the first scenario the nurse sets the agenda and does not allow the patient to participate in formulating goals or to determine the path to take to attain those goals. There were many opportunities to provide information the patient may need or explore some of the barriers that keep this patient from healthy behaviors. The nurse acts as the expert and does not fully assess what the patient knows. Patients need to be allowed to express their needs and help set their personal goals because they are, in fact, the expert in regards to their personal life. They have the answers within them, and it is the nurse's role to help them to find those answers. The patient is clearly overwhelmed and resistant to any suggestions offered by the nurse. If the nurse was more in tune with the patient's needs, he may have recognized the need to step back and take simple steps.

In the second scenario the nurse is more respectful and takes the time to assess how the patient is feeling and what the priorities are in regaining some physical abilities. Instead of the nurse giving instructions, he looks to the patient for the answers based on the premise that the patient is the one that holds all the answers. Essentially, the patient came up with the goal and the steps to take to attain the goal. There is progression from resistance to ambivalence to verbalizing change talk. The nurse offers positive reinforcement for setting an attainable goal and expresses confidence in the patient. This helps boost the patient's feelings of self-efficacy when she feels someone believes in her and believes in her ability to be successful. Clearly, the interaction utilizing motivational interviewing is more effective in promoting behavior change.

Case Study 3

The patient has a history of dyslipidemia. Recent lab work was obtained to determine cholesterol levels.

Interaction Without Motivational Interviewing

> Nurse: Good afternoon. I see you are here to review the blood work you had done last week.
>
> Patient: Yes, that's true.
>
> Nurse: It looks like your total cholesterol and triglycerides are higher. How do you think that happened?
>
> Patient: I don't know.
>
> Nurse: You really need to change your diet. You need to eat low fat, low cholesterol and high fiber foods.
>
> Patient: I have been trying to watch the fat, but I didn't know about the fiber.
>
> Nurse: Well you need more fiber. That will help your heart.
>
> Patient: Okay.
>
> Nurse: You should also be working on exercise to bring the cholesterol levels down. I would recommend at least 4 days a week to get some activity.

Patient: I see.

Nurse: When you come back in a month, I want to see what you are eating and how much exercise you are getting, so please bring a record in for me.

Patient: Okay.

Motivational Interviewing Interaction

Nurse: Good afternoon. I understand you are here today to follow up on your blood work. Did you have any concerns or anything you would like to talk about before looking at the lab results?

Patient: Well, I already know the cholesterol level is still too high. I have been walking three to four times a week, but I have such a hard time with the diet.

Nurse: Tell me about that.

Patient: I love to eat. It's that simple. And that's what you people want to talk about every time I come in here. I just can't do what you ask me to do. (Resistance)

Nurse: I am not here to give you orders. What I would like to do is talk with you about what works or doesn't work for you. I'm here to support you in your efforts to manage the high cholesterol levels.

Patient: Thank you. Like I said the exercise is going pretty well. I actually like going for a walk and look forward to it.

Nurse: There is pleasure, as well as physical benefit, from the walks you take.

Patient: I guess you could say that. My wife and I go on this trail near our house and it's nice to take the dog to walk there, also.

Nurse: That's great. Earlier I mentioned that we have your blood work here and I was wondering if you would like to review that with me.

Patient: I really don't understand the numbers. Just tell me if it's any worse.

Nurse: Would you like me to explain them to you?

Patient: Sure, that might help.

Nurse: The total cholesterol is up a little from the last time, and this gives us a broad picture of how much cholesterol is in your system. The triglycerides went up a few points, too. This is a portion of the cholesterol panel that represents the fat from our food. The good and the bad cholesterol both remained the same. This is the LDL, or **low-density lipoprotein**, and HDL, or **high-density lipoprotein**, and what they do is carry the fat through the bloodstream. You want the LDL to be low and the HDL to be high. What are your thoughts about that?

Patient: Thank you. I think I understand that better now. But like I said, I know the food has a lot to do with it, but I just don't want to eat food that has no taste!

Nurse: You believe that all foods that are healthy for you will not taste good.

Patient: I didn't say that. I have found a few things that are whole grain that taste pretty good.

Nurse: So, you have improved your nutrition.

Patient: We've tried a few things, but I'm not putting all my effort into it.

Nurse: (silence)

Patient: I have too many other things to deal with and my focus has been on the exercise. It is just too much to try to change everything all at once. (Ambivalence)

Nurse: On one hand, you know what you need to do differently to improve your cholesterol levels and decrease your heart disease risks. On the other hand, you are overwhelmed by many other things in your life and are working on activity and nutrition a little at a time because you want to improve your health.

Patient: Yes, I do want to improve my health. I have family I want to stick around for. I just need to work on one goal at a time and it just happens to be the exercise. (Change talk)

Nurse: You should be proud of all the effort you have put into the exercise and the changes you have made in nutrition. Small steps are what bring us to rewards in the end.

Patient: Thank you. It hasn't been easy, but I know I don't want to have a heart attack.

Nurse: I'm confident that as you continue to set small goals for yourself, you will accomplish them and find a healthier lifestyle that works for you.

Discussion

The previous two scenarios look at the difference between interactions without and with the use of motivational interviewing. In the first scenario the patient is not participating in the conversation. The patient is actually put on the defensive by the accusatory statements made by the nurse. Body language and tone of voice could give this interaction a different perspective, but the information provided for this interaction does not give a sense that the nurse and patient are working as a team. This is not a partnership but a relationship where the nurse is superior and the patient is inferior. This goes against the basic premise of motivational interviewing. The patient becomes more passive throughout the interaction. The nurse gives orders as to what needs to be done and what her expectations are for the patient.

In the second scenario there is a partnership. The nurse and patient are working together to meet a common goal: improving the overall health and well-being of the patient. The nurse takes the time to listen and understand the patient's perspective and what drives the patient or may hold the patient back. You can note the use of reflections, both simple and complex. Silence has also been used to encourage patient interaction. Appropriate use of praise propels the momentum the patient has toward achieving his or her goal.

PRACTICE TOOLS (FIGURE 6-2)

1. Recognize the patient as an individual with a cardiovascular deficit or risk for cardiovascular disease. Often, the focus of teaching or goal setting is on issues such as weight loss, exercise, nutrition, and smoking cessation.

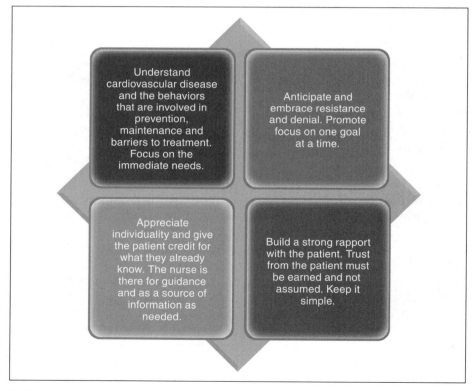

Figure 6-2   Practice Tools

Proper communication will help unearth additional topics that arise from the patient's concerns, which are sometimes indirectly related. For example, the patient may be reluctant to exercise because his or her father was very active and suffered multiple heart attacks that led to his death. A fear of that happening to the patient is a barrier. Or you may find the patient is working so hard to lose weight he or she is going too far in the other direction and not taking in enough calories. This can cause additional problems the patient may not foresee without the therapeutic relationship with the nurse. The goal of the therapeutic interaction is to focus on the patient's immediate needs so he or she can attain goals.

2. Not only should we anticipate resistance and denial of severity of cardiovascular disease, but we should embrace it. Again, many symptoms are silent and that makes it difficult to face the reality and gravity of the illness. Cardiovascular disease is highly preventable, and many negative behaviors can contribute. It is important to recognize the difficulty in changing multiple behaviors concurrently, and one behavior should be addressed at a time to increase the probability for success.

3. Give the patient credit for what he or she does know. This requires the nurse to explore what the patient knows. Without this thorough examination, the nurse can make assumptions based on personal experience and understanding of a particular cardiovascular disease. Appreciate the patient's individuality. The patient has his or her own agenda, and we need to foster growth by allowing the patient to work toward his or her personal goals and be available to provide information when necessary. Gentle guidance will assist the patient to explore his or her own ambivalence and move through the stages of resistance to the point of clarity and beginning of change.

4. Keep it simple. The patient is often stressed and overwhelmed when dealing with a chronic disease such as cardiovascular disease. Many fears and misunderstandings will complicate behavior change. Be sure to encourage the patient to explore those fears. The nurse will need to remain nonjudgmental to maintain a rapport and open communication with the patient. A patient's trust is not a guarantee. It is something the nurse must earn and work to maintain. One research study actually supported focusing on changing multiple behaviors (Kalra & Roitman, 2008). More research is needed to support this theory. As we grow into motivational interviewing, we can gain the skills necessary to potentially focus on more than one behavior at a time.

5. Use your resources:
   • American Heart Association
   • **American Diabetes Association**

- **National Heart, Lung, and Blood Institute**
- American Stroke Association
- **American College of Cardiology**

TAKE-AWAY POINTS

1. Cardiovascular disease is one of the leading causes of mortality in our country. It should be included in every health prevention encounter because many factors that lead to this devastating disease can be prevented.
2. Research has demonstrated that there is a place for motivational interviewing in the health care of those suffering from cardiovascular disease.
3. To achieve the most successful results, recognize the ambivalence the cardiac patient has when weighing the risks and benefits of forgoing treatment and participating in treatment.
4. Be attuned to the change talk when the cardiovascular patient is ready to move towards behavior change and improve his or her cardiac health or decrease his or her risk factors for cardiovascular disease.
5. Be supportive of the patient's thoughts and emotions surrounding cardiovascular disease, in addition to the goals the patient has set.

SUMMARY

The cardiovascular patient has a number of behaviors that can and often need to be changed to improve health and decrease risk factors. The nurse's role is to encourage change in the face of ambivalence. Recognizing the emotional barriers for these particular patients, such as fear, anger, sadness, and denial, is very important. It is also essential to stay attuned to the possible physical barriers that can prevent movement toward cardiac health. Motivational interviewing is an essential tool for the nurse to use when working with the cardiovascular patient.

REFERENCES

American Heart Association. (2009). *Heart disease & stroke statistics—2009 update.* Dallas, Texas: American Heart Association.

Brodie, D., Inoue, A., & Shaw, D. (2008). Motivational interviewing to change quality of life for people with chronic heart failure: A randomized controlled trial. *International Journal of Nursing Studies, 45*(4), 489–500.

CDC. (2009). Heart disease and stroke prevention: Addressing the nation's leading killers, at a glance 2009. Retrieved June 10, 2009, from http://www.cdc.gov/need php/publications/AAG/dhdsp.htm.

Everett, B., Davidson, P., Sheerin, N., Salamonson, Y., & DiGiacomo, M. (2008). Pragmatic insights into a nurse-delivered motivational interviewing intervention in the outpatient cardiac rehabilitation setting. *Journal of Cardiopulmonary Rehabilitation and Prevention, 28*(1), 61–64.

Gatewood, J., Litchfield, R., Ryan, S., Myers Geadelmann, J., Pendergast, J., & Ullom, K. (2008). Perceived barriers to community-based health promotion program participation. *American Journal of Health Behavior, 32*(3), 260–271.

Jaarsma, T., Halfens, R., Tan, F., Abu-Saad, H., Dracup, K., & Diederiks, J. (2000). Self-care and quality of life in patients with advanced heart failure: The effect of a supportive educational intervention. *Heart & Lung: The Journal of Acute and Critical Care, 29*(5), 319–330.

Kalra, S., & Roitman, J. (2008). Simultaneous vs sequential counseling for multiple behavior change. *Journal of Cardiopulmonary Rehabilitation and Prevention, 28*(1), 74–75.

Kreman, R., Yates, B., Agrawal, S., Fiandt, K., Briner, W., & Shurmur, S. (2006). The effects of motivational interviewing on physiological outcomes. *Applied Nursing Research, 19*, 167–170.

National Center for Health Statistics. (2009). *Health, United States, 2008* (pp. 9–17). Hyattsville, MD: U.S. Department of Health and Human Services, Centers for Disease Control and Prevention.

Paul, S., & Sneed, N. (2004). Strategies for behavior change in patients with heart failure. *American Journal of Critical Care, 13*(4), 305–313.

CHAPTER 7

Motivational Interviewing in Endocrine Disease

INTRODUCTION

Endocrine disorders encompass a variety of pathologies. **Type 1** and **type 2 diabetes** are the most well-known diseases from this group of disorders. The endocrine disorders include **hyperthyroidism, hypothyroidism, growth hormone deficiency, polycystic ovary syndrome (PCOS), metabolic syndrome, parathyroid**

disorders, osteoporosis, and a variety of metabolic disorders that are often rare. Of all these disorders, diabetes is most publicized.

Thyroid disease is important to look at because if left untreated it can affect the cardiovascular and musculoskeletal systems and possibly lead to death. Thyroid disease affects 27 million Americans, and half are undiagnosed. More women than men are afflicted. People with diabetes can develop thyroid disorders at a rate of 15-20% in comparison with 4.5% of the general population (see www.medem.com/medlib/print/ZZZNIEIUKIE).

Growth disorders affect children and adults. Too much growth hormone is not very common, affecting less than 100 children and approximately 60 adults for every million Americans. The data on the prevalence of growth hormone deficiency are conflicting, ranging from 1 in 3,500 to 10,000 children. Adult-onset growth hormone deficiency is also unclear. A total of 35,000 people in the United States have growth hormone deficiency, with 6,000 new cases per year (see www.hormone.org/Growth/overview.cfm).

PCOS affects 7-10% of women of childbearing age. "Polycystic ovary syndrome is one of the most common endocrine disorders affecting women across the lifespan" (Baldwin & Witchel, 2006, p. 894). This is a combination of symptoms resulting from an imbalance of androgen hormones. Females who suffer with PCOS are also at an increased risk for diabetes, heart disease, infertility, depression, and some forms of cancer. There are many opportunities for motivational interviewing with this population (see www.hormone.org/Polycystic/overview.cfm).

Hyperparathyroidism, or overactive parathyroid, affects approximately 100,000 American adults. **Addison's disease** and Cushing's syndrome involve the adrenal glands and are a rare occurrence (see www.rwjuh.edu/health_information/adult_endocrin_stats.html). Metabolic disorders are also less common but deserve to be mentioned because they often have a devastating effect on those afflicted and those caring for them because of their disabilities.

The **American Diabetes Association** published a variety of statistics on their Web site. Eight percent of the population has diabetes, and this statistic includes children and adults. What is interesting is that 5.7 million remain undiagnosed. There are 57 million additional people with prediabetes, having demonstrated elevated insulin levels or decreased glucose tolerance. In 2007, $174 billion total was spent on diabetes. The costs are astronomical and include the cost of disability, complications, direct, and indirect care. Diabetes is the fifth leading cause of death, and the incidence has been increasing since 1987 (see www.diabetes.org/diabetes-statistics.jsp).

There is a significant focus on diabetes self-management. **Diabetes self-management education** is a worthwhile investment because it decreases the cost of treatment and risk of complications and improves self-efficacy. Diabetes management is highly dependent on patient involvement in his or her care (Boren et al., 2009). The **American Association of Diabetes Educators** provides seven guidelines for self-management, called the AADE7. This is a framework for self-care behaviors that promote patient involvement in seven areas of health (Figure 7-1). This framework is based on the premise that patients who are involved in their care are more successful. This organization does not claim to use motivational interviewing per se, but the education and management is central to empowering the patient. The belief is that the nurse provides the proper tools and the patient can then make informed choices when making healthcare decisions (see www.diabeteseducator.org/ProfessionalResources/AADE7/).

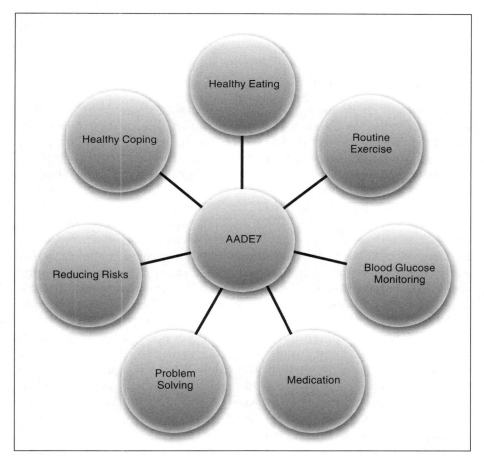

Figure 7-1   Diabetes Self Management

Source: Adapted from http://www.diabeteseducator.org/ProfessionalResources/AADE7/

Healthy People 2010 specifically designates diabetes as a focus area. We have come a long way in managing diabetes and promoting self-management, but with so many comorbidities and the effects of diabetes on our healthcare system, the focus remains strong. Many aspects of diabetes management are also included in the Healthy People 2010 focus areas:

- Chronic kidney disease
- Heart disease and stroke
- Nutrition and overweight
- Physical activity and fitness
- Tobacco use

Improving each of these areas will positively impact the health of our diabetes population, who make up 8% of our total population (see www.healthypeople. gov/About/hpfact.htm).

CHALLENGES IN ENDOCRINE DISORDERS

There are many challenges in managing any one of the many endocrine disorders. Some endocrine disorders, such as Cushing's disease, can be difficult to diagnose. The presentation of clinical symptoms may be vague, many symptoms are related to comorbidities, or the endocrine disorder becomes one of many in the provider's differential. Many of the disorders can also be linked to one another, such as the increased risk for glaucoma with thyroid disease or the increased risk for diabetes with PCOS or metabolic syndrome (Haigh, 2008; Kalvaitis, 2008; Milone, 2008). Some endocrine disorders require us to delve into discussions regarding patients' hormones, including sex hormones. This is an uncomfortable, but a necessary, topic for many people. For example, a woman with hirsutism may have significant emotional issues regarding her personal appearance and decrease in self-esteem as a result. Every disorder requires a behavior to manage it. And because we are not perfect, there is likely to be some behavior that needs to be changed to achieve our highest potential.

Being diagnosed with an endocrine disorder is one thing. It is another to come to understand it and then be able to self-manage some, if not all, aspects of treatment. Diabetes is one disorder that is highly self-manageable. "More than 95% of diabetes care is done by the patient and diabetes self-management education is the cornerstone of care for individuals with diabetes" (Bazata, Robinson, Fox, & Grandy, 2008, p. 1026). Diabetes self-management education is built right into the treatment plan. The self-management can be complicated, and there are many barriers that can interfere—some created by the diabetes. Some of the aspects of diabetes self-management education include nutrition, exercise, medication, foot care, and eye care. Some of the complications of diabetes include blindness, kidney failure, chronic skin ulcers, heart disease, and gastroparesis. Heart disease, blindness, taking medication, foot care, and nutrition can all impact success with exercise. Imagine the number of topics that could come up in the conversation. Determining the focus may be difficult for the patient who is overwhelmed.

A variety of body systems can be affected by endocrine disorders, and the focus of the interaction may require more work to ascertain. What the patient sees as the problem may be completely different from what the nurse may suspect or assume is the issue. It may be more difficult for the nurse to step back and not take on the expert role. We are accustomed to discharge papers that provide a list of patient instructions. There was a time when we would just read off the instructions and educate only if patients had questions. To be more effective we need to take advantage of this time to provide understanding, support, and encouragement as well as education. The nurse and patient must assume a corelationship.

Another challenge is the complexity of the disorders, making treatment more complicated and difficult for the patient to follow through. The ambivalence may be profound. Consider the teenager with type 1 diabetes who has to self-administer injections. He or she is likely to hate the injections while recognizing the importance of taking them. The teenager does not want to do it but feels he or she has no choice.

There may not be a desire to change. The nurse may see the patient is not taking the medication and feels responsible for ensuring the patient complies. This aspect of motivational interviewing, that the patient has the ability to make his or her own choices, even if it is not the healthiest choice, can be challenging to grasp. The patient may choose not to take the medication because of the side effects. To that patient the risks outweigh the benefits. Helping the patient to explore other options, rather than force the perspective that the medication is necessary, enhances the nurse–patient relationship and allows the patient to be more self-efficacious. "The theory of psychological reactance predicts an increase in the rate and attractiveness of a 'problem' behavior if a person perceives that his or her personal freedom is being infringed or challenged" (Miller & Rollnick, 2002, p. 18). To increase the possibility of a positive behavior change, the nurse must encourage patients to determine the negative behaviors they believe they can change.

BENEFITS OF SELF-MANAGEMENT

One benefit of self-management in endocrine disorders is that the patient is making the decisions and creating attainable personal goals instead of the nurse reading over rote instructions. The nurse aids in the process of change instead of attempting to force the change. More research is necessary to evaluate the benefits of self-management in other areas aside from diabetes. Much is left to be discovered about the effectiveness of motivational interviewing in endocrine disorders other than diabetes. Diabetes is one area that has been studied a number of times.

In one particular study, motivational interviewing was used as an adjunct to a group weight loss program. The study included 217 women with type 2 diabetes and overweight. The experimental group participated in the weight loss program and received six motivational interviewing sessions. Follow-up occurred at 3, 6, 12, and 18 months. The results of this study favored the use of motivational interviewing to increase weight loss, to increase success of weight maintenance, and to lower **hemoglobin A_{Ic}** levels (3-month glucose average). This is an obvious benefit to the diabetes community (Deangelis, 2007). Upcoming studies will utilize the **average blood glucose** to take the place of the hemoglobin A_{Ic} level.

Another study "evaluated whether health knowledge, attitudes, and behaviors of individuals with type 1 (T1DM) or type 2 (T2DM) diabetes mellitus and those at high or low risk of T2DM were reflected in healthy behaviors and whether these attributes differed for T2DM respondents who did or did not see a health educator" (Bazata et al., 2008, p. 1025). The **SHIELD study** (The Study to Help Improve Early evaluation and management of risk factors Leading to Diabetes) is a longitudinal study that began in 2004. The study is self-reported and evaluates unmet medical needs among other things. The focus is determination of behavior change for those who met with a dietitian or health educator versus those who did not. Results of this study found that people know what they need to do to manage diabetes and their risk factors but have not followed through with behavior change. "Interaction with health educators and patient-empowering support may improve the transition to behavior change" (Bazata et al., 2008, p. 1026). Motivational interviewing accomplishes this task.

Conversation maps are tools designed to promote open discussions that allow the patient to reflect and explore feelings and experiences living with diabetes. These maps were created and first used in Canada in 2005. The success of these maps has encouraged the American Diabetes Association to bring the maps to the United States to promote self-efficacy and potentially behavior change. This tool allows patients to communicate with others who have faced similar challenges and to gain insight to personal behaviors and help create attainable goals. They are patient centered and promote educational opportunities in a nonthreatening atmosphere. All those who participate are experts and allow the nurse to be supportive rather than directive (Belton, 2008).

CASE STUDIES

The following are case studies for nurse–patient interactions using both non-motivational interviewing techniques and motivational interviewing tactics. Compare the effect on promoting behavior change for each scenario.

Case Study 1

A 15-year-old boy with delayed puberty is in the office to discuss hormone therapy. The parent wants this therapy initiated, yet the adolescent is resistant.

Interaction Without Motivational Interviewing

> Nurse: Good morning. How are you today?
>
> Patient: I guess I'm doing okay.
>
> Nurse: Good. I understand you are here today to talk about starting hormone therapy. Is that correct?
>
> Patient: I guess so. My mother wants me to do it, but I don't.
>
> Nurse: At your age your mother knows best. Now let's get started and I'll show you how to administer the injections.
>
> Patient: (silent)
>
> Nurse: Your doctor will prescribe a dose. I'm going to show you how to draw up 5 cc of medication and then I want you to practice. (Nurse demonstrates procedure.)
>
> Patient: (silent)
>
> Nurse: Very good. Now I'm going to show you how to administer an injection, and I want you to show me how to do it. (Nurse demonstrates procedure.)
>
> Patient: (silent)
>
> Nurse: Do you have any questions?
>
> Patient: No.
>
> Nurse: You should be all set now. Good luck.

Motivational Interviewing Interaction

> Nurse: Good morning. How are you doing today?
>
> Patient: I'm okay, I guess.
>
> Nurse: You don't sound too sure about that.
>
> Patient: Well, I know I'm here to start on the hormone therapy and I'm not sure I want to do it. (Ambivalence)

Nurse: Tell me your thoughts on this.

Patient: My mom really wants me to do this. And I agree that it would help me fit in better with my classmates, but I like me the way I am. I don't want to take hormones. (Resistance)

Nurse: You feel that taking the hormone therapy will change you.

Patient: Maybe it will.

Nurse: Why do you think your mother wants you to do this?

Patient: She tells me that I'm not normal looking and that is why I don't have friends or a girlfriend.

Nurse: (silence)

Patient: She's right. I don't look normal and I hate that she looks at me like I'm a freak. I'm not a freak.

Nurse: No, you are not. You already feel different and it hurts that your mother spoke the words that you feel.

Patient: That's just it. Maybe it's the whole control thing. I don't want my mother to tell me what I need to do. I am old enough to make my own decisions.

Nurse: I agree. Could you share with me your thoughts about what are the positive and negative points of doing hormone therapy?

Patient: Well, the good part would be that I would fit in and I might feel better about how I look, but at the same time, I would be giving my mother control.

Nurse: I'm curious what is good or bad about not using hormone therapy.

Patient: The good part would be that I have control over my own body, but the bad part would be that I may not grow up physically.

Nurse: Not having the physical characteristics typical of one's age can be challenging and contribute to other problems.

Patient: I don't think people would take me as seriously if I don't look my age.

Nurse: (silence)

Patient: I also know that it could ultimately affect my ability to have kids. I don't want any right now, but I may want to be a dad someday. (Change talk)

Nurse: You have excellent insight to the pros and cons of this treatment. I am confident that you will choose the best path for you.

Patient: Thank you. You have helped me to see that it is important to me to receive the therapy, even if it is for different reasons than my mother wants.

Discussion

The first scenario demonstrated a teaching session, not an interactive communication between nurse and patient. The nurse acted as the expert and dismissed the patient's feelings and concerns about starting hormone therapy. Although the patient is an adolescent, he needs to be included in the discussion about treatment. In this scenario the nurse did most of the talking, with no reflections or exploration of the patient's level of understanding or concerns about hormone therapy. The nurse was clearly not actively listening or may have delved into the patient's first statement, exploring the patient's emotions regarding this visit.

The second scenario has more effective results in regards to the patient's perspective on hormone therapy. By exploring the patient's perspective, the nurse was better able to gently guide the patient through the decision-making process. The nurse respected the patient as she would an adult. She respected the patient's thoughts, values, and perspective. The patient was able to come to a conclusion independent of the parent. Another scenario may include the parent. In this scenario the nurse did not feed into the negative statements, otherwise the conversation could have been about the patient's relationship with the parent. The nurse effectively kept the focus on the patient and what his thoughts were about treatment. This was a successful motivational interviewing encounter.

Case Study 2

A 24-year-old woman with PCOS has increased her weight by 10 pounds in the past 3 months. She is not taking the Metformin that was prescribed. She is not following any of the recommendations from the provider.

Interaction Without Motivational Interviewing

Nurse: Good afternoon. How are you doing?

Patient: I could be better. I saw that I had gained 10 pounds.

Nurse: You really need to lose weight. I also see you are not taking the Metformin your doctor prescribed.

Patient: No, you're right.

Nurse: The doctor ordered it to help with insulin sensitivity. This helps to make sure your body uses the food you eat appropriately. You don't want to develop diabetes, too.

Patient: I couldn't eat right, and I was having so many stomach problems that I just couldn't keep taking it.

Nurse: Oh. Those side effects go away. You should go back on the medication.

Patient: I can't take it. I tried.

Nurse: You didn't give it enough time. Start taking it again tomorrow morning.

Patient: Okay.

Motivational Interviewing Interaction

Nurse: Good afternoon. How are you doing?

Patient: I'm doing well. Thanks.

Nurse: I thought we could talk about the doctor's recommendations for treatment of your PCOS, but first I'm hoping to hear from you if you have anything you would like to talk about.

Patient: Well, I'm really upset about the weight gain.

Nurse: You aren't happy with your weight.

Patient: Not at all. I tried to do what the doctor told me about eating healthy and exercising and was doing pretty well for a couple weeks, but then I had an injury and just haven't gotten back into the routine. I'm just frustrated and I can't do it. (Resistance)

Nurse: You had a great start and should be proud of that accomplishment. I'm sorry to hear about your injury. It can be very difficult to get back into a routine after a disruption. Do you have any thoughts on how you might go about that?

Patient: I have thought about it and considered some starting dates and can write it on the calendar as if it is an appointment I have to keep.

Nurse: You want to get started again, but at the same time you look at it as an obligation and not something you really want to do.

Patient: You could say that. I just can't get to a point of thinking that this is something I have to keep up forever. It makes it harder to get through one session of exercise.

Nurse: You are not alone. Many people go through a difficult time getting started and maintaining an exercise routine. I would love to hear what you have tried so far.

Patient: I have tried an aerobics class, kick boxing class, and went for walks. I liked the idea of the class setting but want something at a slower pace than aerobics. If I could find something I could enjoy, it might work better. (Ambivalence)

Nurse: Would you mind me sharing with you some ideas I have heard from other patients in your situation?

Patient: I would appreciate it.

Nurse: I have heard many people that haven't spent a lot of time exercising or participating in sports say that they enjoy things like water aerobics and yoga. Both are done in a class and are lower impact than the cardio aerobics taught in the gyms.

Patient: I think I'll look into those. They both sound like I might enjoy them and it can't hurt to try. (Change talk)

Discussion

In the first scenario the nurse was authoritarian and did not listen to what the patient was saying. Eventually, the patient gave up and became passive. The nurse actually sounded very demanding and stayed in the expert role. The patient attempted to exert some personal stake in her own health and treatment. The nurse assumed that the benefits of taking Metformin outweighed the risks, including side effects. The nurse and patient were not in the same place during this conversation.

The second scenario demonstrates the use of motivational interviewing. Compared with the first interaction, the nurse let the patient guide the way and focus on what would help make this successful for the patient. Assumptions were not made in regards to what was important to the patient. The nurse did not demand change. The nurse recognized that the patient is the one who is going through the process and the nurse's role is that of support. The nurse remained nonjudgmental and walked beside the patient.

Case Study 3

A 62-year-old patient has a 6-year history of type 2 diabetes. The level of control has been variable since diagnosis. The patient has a variety of physical barriers to successful self-management.

Interaction Without Motivational Interviewing

Nurse: Good morning. I just looked over your blood glucose readings for the past 2 weeks and the numbers are quite scattered.

Patient: I know. I have been trying so hard, but I just can't get control.

Nurse: Getting control over your blood glucose is important to prevent long-term complications. It also helps you to feel better.

Patient: Well, I haven't been feeling very well.

Nurse: Let's look at your blood glucose together. I'm sure we can come up with a way to get better control.

Patient: Okay.

Nurse: I recommend you eat and take your medication at the same time each day. The more consistent you are, the better the numbers you will see. Make sure you eat similar meals from day to day, also. For example, eat one slice of toast with a banana one day, and the next day, eat a small muffin with some grapes.

Patient: I try to keep on schedule, but my vision is bad and I don't know if I always read the clock right. And if my daughter doesn't get a chance to draw up all my insulin for me, I might miss some doses.

Nurse: Oh, you can't miss any doses of insulin, or that will definitely cause your blood glucose to be elevated.

Patient: I do the best I can, but it's not easy.

Nurse: I'm sure it isn't easy, but it is essential to keeping you healthy and not having any more complications occur.

Patient: I really don't know how I can fix some of these problems. I live alone and my daughter lives an hour away. She can only come visit every couple of weeks.

Nurse: We will set up for a nurse to come to your home to help then. How is that?

Motivational Interviewing Interaction

Nurse: Good morning. How have you been?

Patient: The same as always. My blood sugar is all over the place.

Nurse: Some people strive for perfection, and others are more accepting of the wide fluctuations that can occur with the blood glucose. Would you consider yourself at one of those extremes or somewhere in between?

Patient: I think I would be somewhere in between. I don't expect perfection, but I'm also not happy with the ups and downs of my blood sugar.

Nurse: You aren't happy with your blood glucose levels, but at the same time you are not looking to have perfect numbers, either. Would you like to talk about ways to improve your control?

Patient: I have done everything I can. My vision is bad and that makes it hard to draw up my own insulin. I can't cook anymore because I'm afraid I may burn myself. My daughter tries to help, but she lives an hour away and can only come visit every few weeks. I'm not asking her to help anymore than she already has. I will just keep going like I am going. (Resistance)

Nurse: Your daughter must love you very much to come help out when she can.

Patient: Oh she does. She works so hard and worries about me all the time. I don't want her worrying. If I could be more independent, she wouldn't have to worry as much. It's so hard to deal with the blindness, but there should be some way to do things on my own. (Ambivalence)

Nurse: There are many tools to help people in your situation. If you are interested, I would be happy to talk with you about those tools.

Patient: Sure. If you have ideas, that would be helpful.

Nurse: Other patients I have worked with have found talking glucose meters to be helpful in monitoring the blood glucose. There are watches that can be set to alarm at meal or medication times. One tool I think would be particularly helpful would be the insulin pen. The insulin is in the pen and only the needle needs to be replaced. The dosage can be determined by listening to the clicking sound and counting up to the dose you need. They are easy to inject and all you have to do is push a button.

Patient: I think I'd like to try the insulin pen. Then my daughter doesn't have to drive here to draw up my insulin ahead of time. (Change talk)

Nurse: We can spend a few moments going over the technique, and I'll give you a demonstration pen to use for practice until you get comfortable with listening and counting the clicks to get the dosage you need.

Patient: Thank you. I appreciate you taking the time to help me.

Discussion

The previous two scenarios revolve around a patient who is looking to gain independence in her diabetes self-management. The interactions vary in the direction the conversations headed, and the result was significantly more positive in the motivational interviewing interaction.

The first scenario reflected the nurse as the expert. The nurse did not explore the patient's barriers to successful self-management. The nurse assumed the patient was simply reluctant to follow through with care recommendations. Patient statements that offered some reasons behind the barriers were disregarded by the nurse. Opportunities to have the patient further investigate her personal barriers were missed. The patient gave information freely, and the nurse did not respond. A strong rapport could not be established from this conversation.

The second scenario demonstrates a more successful flow of conversation. The patient and nurse move together through the stages of resistance, ambivalence, and preparedness to change. The nurse invited the patient to participate and only offered information when the patient got stuck. Permission to ask questions was requested, and information was only provided when the patient was ready to receive it. Just by listening the nurse was able to evoke information about the patient's barriers to treatment. Without that information the nurse could simply assume the patient voluntarily chooses not to participate in treatment. The patient would simply continue living in a manner that put her at risk for complications.

PRACTICE TOOLS (FIGURE 7-2)

1. Recognize the complexity of endocrine disorders and the challenges this brings to the patient who is afflicted. The challenges for the nurse and healthcare providers to fully understand the spectrum of disorders are minimal compared with that of the patient who may be newly diagnosed. Do not assume the patient has a thorough understanding of what is happening inside his or her body. Recognizing when behavior modification has a place in treatment is essential. Even when motivational interviewing is not likely to help, the nurse should always use some of the tactics, such as being empathetic, having a nonjudgmental attitude, and showing respect for personal choices.

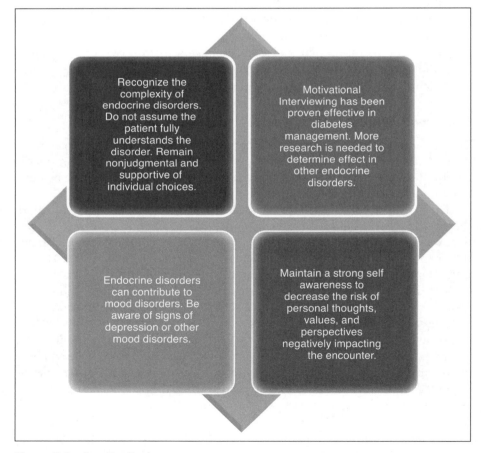

Figure 7-2   Practice Tools

2. Diabetes is the most common endocrine disorder that has proven to be effectively managed with motivational interviewing interactions. More studies are necessary to determine the effectiveness of motivational interviewing in the care of people with other endocrine disorders. The American Association of Diabetes Educators has dedicated a significant amount of time and energy into creating guidelines for the practitioner to use when interacting with patients to improve the outcomes of behavior change.
3. There is a strong emotional current for those diagnosed with an endocrine disorder. The disorder itself may cause mood swings that leave the patient feeling out of control. The effects of the illness or a precipitating factor of weight gain can have a lasting effect on self-esteem. For patients whose physical attributes are changed or are perceived as abnormal, the disorder also has an effect on how they feel about themselves. Remaining nonjudgmental and gaining the trust of the patient is vital to a therapeutic relationship. Be aware of signs of depression for this population.
4. The nurse should have a strong self-awareness, paying attention to reflection of personal views, body language, tone of voice, and general portrayal of judgment. How the patient perceives the nurse's involvement in the conversation predicts the outcome. Forming a therapeutic relationship is essential to the patient feeling at ease to share thoughts and concerns about his or her disorder.
5. Take advantage of the resources available:
   - American Association of Diabetes Educators
   - American Diabetes Association
   - **American Association of Clinical Endocrinologists**
   - American Thyroid Association
   - Endocrine Society
   - The Hormone Foundation
   - Human Growth Foundation
   - National Organization for Rare Disorders
   - National Endocrine and Metabolic Disease Information Service

TAKE-AWAY POINTS

1. Endocrine disorders affect a large portion of our population. Some disorders are quite rare, but thyroid disease and diabetes are more common. Combined with the comorbidities, the endocrine disorders encompass a vast majority of our population.
2. Motivational interviewing has been proven effective in the management of patients with type 1 and type 2 diabetes and chronic illness in general. Ongoing research will help to determine its use in other endocrine disorders.

3. The AADE7 helps to guide the practice of nurse educators and encompasses many of the motivational interviewing techniques. This can be used with patients who suffer other endocrine disorders with little modification, less the blood glucose monitoring.
4. Be aware that not all patients want to change and may be happy with status quo. Part of motivational interviewing embraces the patient's choice not to make a change.
5. Incorporation of mental health resources may be beneficial to those struggling with the emotional aspects of their disorder.

SUMMARY

Patients with disorders of the endocrine system can benefit from motivational interviewing interventions. The nurse can offer the necessary tools to help promote successful behavior change. Several endocrine disorders are linked to obesity, and we have seen evidence of motivational interviewing being effective when approaching nutrition and exercise. Because diabetes is highly self-managed, there has been more discussion and research in this area. Healthy People 2010 urges us to focus on several areas that are tied into precipitating factors, side effects, and comorbidities of endocrine disorders.

REFERENCES

Baldwin, C., & Witchel, S. (2006). Polycystic ovary syndrome. *Pediatric Annals, 35*(12), 888–896.

Bazata, D., Robinson, J., Fox, K., & Grandy, S. (2008). Affecting behavior change in individuals with diabetes: Findings from the study to help improve early evaluation and management of risk factors leading to diabetes (SHIELD). *The Diabetes Educator, 34*(6), 1025–1036.

Belton, A. (2008). Conversation maps in Canada: The first 2 years. *Diabetes Spectrum, 21*(2), 139–142.

Boren, S., Fitzner, K., Panhalkar, P., & Specker, J. (2009). Costs and benefits associated with diabetes education: A review of the literature. *The Diabetes Educator, 35*(1), 72–96.

Deangelis, T. (2007). Patient empowerment improves outcomes: Technique that bolsters patient buy-in pays off in reduced weight, lower A_{Ic}'s. *DOC News, 4*(12), 1.

Haigh, C. (2008). Metabolic syndrome was strong predictor of incident diabetes. *Endocrine Today, 6*(20), 15.

Kalvaitis, K. (2008). Thyroid disorder may be a risk factor for developing glaucoma. *Endocrine Today, 6*(21), 24.

Miller, W., & Rollnick, S. (2002). *Motivational Interviewing: Preparing people for change* (2nd ed.). New York: The Guilford Press.

Milone, A. (2008). The difficulties of Cushing's syndrome. *Endocrine Today, 6*(21), 1, 12–14.

CHAPTER 8

Motivational Interviewing in Digestive Health

INTRODUCTION

Gastrointestinal disorders are an important group of disorders that can benefit from the use of motivational interviewing. Many of these disorders are quite common and can be improved, if not eliminated, by behavior change. Both acute and chronic, these illnesses have a significant impact on the health of our nation. The effects are a combination of physical, emotional, social, and financial. The nurse is at the forefront to help the patients improve their lifestyle to decrease risks, manage symptoms, and avoid complications.

Viral gastroenteritis is very common and highly contagious. It is the second most common illness in the United States (see digestive.niddk.nih.gov/ddiseases/pubs/viralgastroenteritis/index.htm). Millions of children and adults have cases of diarrhea each year. Rotavirus has such an impact on our nation's health that we now immunize our children against it. Frequent hand washing is the best way to avoid infection. Hospitalization can occur because of dehydration as a direct result of viral gastroenteritis, driving up our healthcare costs.

On the opposite end of the spectrum is constipation. This is another disorder that arises from the gastrointestinal system. "More than 4 million Americans have frequent constipation, accounting for 2.5 million physician visits a year. . . . Around $725 million is spent on laxative products each year in America" (see digestive.niddk.nih.gov/ddiseases/pubs/constipation/index.htm). Although no long-term complications typically occur with constipation, it is still important to make note of the impact it has on our country. Dietary changes, proper fluid intake, and routine exercise are behaviors that can improve these statistics.

Ulcers, such as peptic ulcers, are also common. "One in 10 Americans develops an ulcer at some time in his or her life" (see digestive.niddk.nih.gov/ddiseases/pubs/hpylori/index.htm). The common cause is the bacteria, *Helicobacter pylori*. Little is known about how *H. pylori* gets into our system, but research is underway to develop an immunization for this disease. Certain behaviors can help improve the symptoms and the outcome of this disease. Nurses may need to promote behavior change in areas such as diet, overuse of over-the-counter medications, avoidance of medications that can worsen symptoms, and following the treatment regimen for *H. pylori*.

Gastroesophageal reflux disease is also quite common. This affects all populations, from infancy to the elderly. When untreated, this can lead to more serious health problems. These complications include bleeding of the stomach lining, strictures of the esophagus, and esophageal cancer, which can be fatal. Given the dire consequences, it is important to recognize the importance of maintaining healthy behaviors and follow through with treatment recommendations. The nurse has an important role in helping the patient to understand and make informed decisions about their daily care (see digestive.niddk.nih.gov/ddiseases/pubs/gerd/index.htm).

Celiac disease is a genetic disorder that interferes with proper absorption of certain proteins found in wheat, rye, and barley. This significantly lessens the food choices available and can affect a child's growth. It can also occur in adults, may be asymptomatic, or can go years before being diagnosed. When improperly treated, it can lead to serious complications such as miscarriage, osteoporosis, liver disease, and intestinal cancer. Over 2 million people are afflicted by this disease in the United States. Patients with this condition make choices each day about their meals and snacks. Outcomes are improved when the patient is given adequate information and makes appropriate choices when meal planning (see digestive.niddk.nih.gov/ddiseases/pubs/celiac/index.htm).

Irritable bowel syndrome is also one of the most common disorders, affecting 20% of the U.S. population. Although not a serious disease with significant long-term complications, it can be very uncomfortable and cause a lot of distress, leading to missed work and inability to leave the home for any length of time due to the symptoms. Stress management and diet can help and are behaviors controlled by the patient (see digestive.niddk.nih.gov/ddiseases/pubs/ibs/index.htm).

Diverticulosis affects 10% of Americans over 40 years of age, and for those older than 60, almost half are afflicted (see digestive.niddk.nih.gov/ddiseases/pubs/diverticulosis/index.htm). Self-management is useful because each person is different in their response to foods and how these foods impact symptoms. Helping the patient to find the best way to manage the dietary aspect of treatment can be done by a nurse or a nutritionist. Making dietary changes is not easy, and motivational interviewing is a tool that can assist in accomplishing this goal.

Hepatitis is a liver disease that can be quite devastating. The three most common forms of viral hepatitis are hepatitis A, B, and C. Hepatitis A is transmitted by the fecal-oral route. In 2006 there were 3,579 new cases of hepatitis A and 4,713 new cases of hepatitis B (see www.cdc.gov/nchs/fastats/hepatits.htm). Hepatitis B and C are transmitted by blood and body fluids and are often considered sexually transmitted. Hepatitis C "accounts for about 15 percent of acute viral hepatitis, 60 to 70 percent of chronic hepatitis, and up to 50 percent of **cirrhosis**, end-stage liver disease, and liver cancer" (see digestive.niddk.nih.gov/ddiseases/pubs/chronichepc/index.htm). There is a high probability that those with acute illness will develop a chronic infection of hepatitis C, increasing the mortality statistics.

Inflammation of the pancreas, or **pancreatitis**, can be acute or chronic. An estimated 210,000 hospitalizations occur each year due to acute pancreatitis. The digestive enzymes become active while still in the pancreas, and when there is inflammation, the enzymes attack the pancreatic tissue, leading to abdominal pain and other symptoms. Pancreatitis is a serious condition that can lead to chronic pain, diabetes, and possible surgery (see digestive.niddk.nih.gov/ddiseases/pubs/pancreatitis/index.htm).

A discussion about the impact that gastrointestinal disorders have in the United States cannot occur without mentioning obesity (see www.cdc.gov/nccdphp/publications/AAG/obesity.htm). One-third of adults and 16% of children are obese. In 2000 the healthcare costs related to obesity were about $117 billion. The comorbidities are

- Coronary heart disease
- Type 2 diabetes
- Hypertension
- Dyslipidemia
- Stroke
- Liver and gallbladder disease
- Sleep apnea
- Osteoarthritis
- Irregular menses/infertility
- Psychosocial issues

Behavior change is the cornerstone to preventing, managing, and preventing long-term complications of obesity.

Healthy People 2010 recognizes the importance of focusing on obesity. Focus areas include nutrition and overweight, physical activity, and fitness. Healthy People 2010 also addresses multiple complications that occur with obesity, such as diabetes and cardiovascular disease, as well as immunizations. Immunizations for rotavirus, hepatitis A, and hepatitis B are available and advance us one step closer to improving the impact of these gastrointestinal viruses in the United States (see www.healthypeople.gov/About/hpfact.htm).

CHALLENGES IN GASTROINTESTINAL DISORDERS

Some gastrointestinal disorders are tied to other issues that can cloud the focus of an encounter. For example, liver disease and pancreatitis can be caused by alcohol abuse. Trying to focus on one without the other may be helpful for some, whereas others may need to see the connection. The nurse may see the direct interaction between alcohol abuse and cirrhosis of the liver, but the patient may be resistant to make that connection. If patients are in denial about the alcohol addiction, they may not be ready to discuss their drinking patterns and how it relates to their disease. When an illness is directly caused by one's actions, it can be difficult for the patient to accept the need to change, and the encounter could be filled with resistance.

Gastrointestinal disorders that require dietary changes can also be challenging. It can be difficult to change eating patterns because of personal preferences, physical inability to do one's own shopping, and financial constraints. Eating healthy can be costly. When people live on a fixed income, it can be difficult to buy things such as fresh fruits and vegetables. Special foods, such as gluten-free foods needed for those with celiac disease, are even more expensive. We can educate on healthy diets, but a patient's perception of his or her personal eating habits may not agree with our perception. With such barriers to behavior change in nutrition, the nurse may struggle with this aspect of the patient's treatment.

Obesity is very complicated and carries a negative stigma because of physical appearance and the health risks that are associated with it. There are many causes of obesity (Figure 8-1). Overeating is not the only contributing factor but tends to be the easiest one for providers to address. It is easy to counsel about healthy nutrition. Some people eat healthy and exercise but still suffer from obesity, so discussing healthy nutrition is not a therapeutic for that population. Finding the source of the obesity problem for each individual can be challenging. Too often assumptions are made and the source is not fully investigated. Patients also have many emotions revolving around their weight, and self-esteem suffers due to unsuccessful attempts at weight loss. Our values can alter our interactions with people who suffer from this condition, and it can be challenging to remain nonjudgmental because we know the health risks involved with obesity. Motivational interviewing provides us with tactics to address the issue in a way that allows the patient to explore his or her thoughts and feelings and make informed decisions, and, hopefully, supports the patient as he or she creates attainable goals to healthier living.

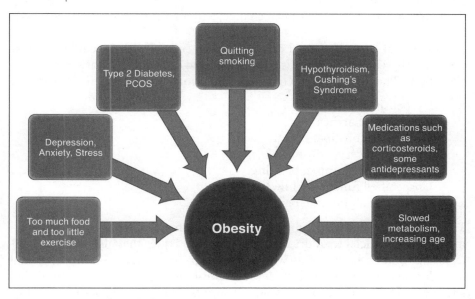

Figure 8-1   Factors Contributing to Obesity

BENEFITS OF SELF-MANAGEMENT

There are numerous lifestyle choices that can help prevent many gastrointestinal disorders. Self-management can help decrease the risk of long-term complications. A variety of lifestyle choices can affect the gastrointestinal system, such as nutrition, alcohol consumption, stress, exercise, medication, and prevention through hand washing and immunization. Motivational interviewing has been found to be effective in many of these areas.

Obesity has been researched more than any other aspect of gastrointestinal health. Although it is seen by some as true disorder, some view it as a symptom. Regardless of that perspective, motivational interviewing can positively impact the obesity statistics in America. Because behavior has a primary role, albeit not the only role, in managing obesity, we need to focus on behaviors that can contribute to this devastating problem. School-based programs have been initiated because our children spend a majority of their time away from home at school. School nurses can have a direct impact on the children who are at risk for or already suffer from obesity. One study found the obesity problem to be only second to drug abuse and violence. This is a clear indication that this is a problem that significantly impacts our healthcare system and we need to address it. Providing options for healthy eating and exercise allow children to begin making choices and become involved in the future of their health (Clark & Slemmons, 2008). "We are not responsible for whether or not they change but for helping them decide if they want to or can change, and if so, how to do so" (Glovsky & Rose, 2007, p. 50).

Functional gastrointestinal disorders often coexist with psychological disorders, such as anxiety, panic disorder, and mood disorders (Guthrie & Thompson, 2002). The following are considered functional gastrointestinal disorders:

- Dyspepsia
- Functional diarrhea
- Functional constipation
- Irritable bowel syndrome
- Functional abdominal bloating
- Unspecified functional bowel disorder
- Functional abdominal pain syndrome

The patient may have difficulty coping that can interfere with overall management. It is beneficial to address the psychosocial issues that also arise. It is interesting to note that patients who suffer from the functional gastrointestinal disorders also have a fairly high level of abuse history. One study found that 44% of patients with gastrointestinal disorders also had a history of sexual or physical abuse (Drossman, Talley, Leserman, Olden, & Barreiro, 1995). Patients with this combination of issues can benefit from motivational interviewing because it can help them gain some self-control. Having some control over their future can help give back what control may have been lost due to abuse. The nurse will need to be aware of the potential barriers related to the comorbidity of psychosocial deficits in this population. The nurse can help the patient explore how to effectively manage the symptoms of the gastrointestinal disorder and promote self-efficacy (Cash, 2005; Drossman et al., 1995; Guthrie & Thompson, 2002).

We recognize that stress has an effect on the gastrointestinal system and can cause other physical problems. Motivational interviewing offers a positive approach to promoting behavior change in relation to stress. Research has been done on the relationship between stress and those suffering from gastrointestinal disorders. There is some suggestion that people with gastrointestinal disorders may actually feel pain more acutely. "Stress can make the existing pain seem even worse" (see www.aarp.org/health/conditions/articles/harvard_the-sensitive-gut_2.html). Controlling stress can actually help gastrointestinal symptoms. Stress management may be a common topic during a motivational interviewing session with a patient afflicted by a gastrointestinal disorder.

CASE STUDIES

The following case studies demonstrate effective and ineffective encounters with patients who have a gastrointestinal disorder. Differences between the two scenarios demonstrate how motivational interviewing can promote behavior change.

Case Study 1

The patient has celiac disease and has been in the emergency room multiple times for gastrointestinal complaints. He is in for a follow-up appointment.

Interaction Without Motivational Interviewing

Nurse: Good morning. How are you doing?

Patient: I'm pretty good now.

Nurse: I see you are here today because you were in the emergency room again.

Patient: I have tried to follow the diet. I'm tired of feeling sick all the time, but I just can't do it.

Nurse: I'm going to give you a list of gluten-free foods and let's go over them to see what we can do about your diet.

Patient: We've gone over this before. I know what foods are gluten free and what to look for on the food labels.

Nurse: Then I don't understand what the problem is. Following that diet is the only way you are going to feel well.

Patient: (silent)

Nurse: What I would like to have you do is try to follow the gluten-free diet for 1 week. Keep a food diary so we can see where you could do better.

Patient: Okay.

Nurse: I'm sure you'll feel better once you start following the gluten-free diet.

Patient: (silent)

Motivational Interviewing Interaction

Nurse: Good morning. How are you doing?

Patient: I'm pretty good today.

Nurse: I see you were in the emergency room again. What can you tell me about that?

Patient: I got sick again. I am so tired of not feeling good. I don't want to even deal with celiac disease. (Resistance)

Nurse: It can be very frustrating when you feel so sick all the time.

Patient: It is. I did so well for awhile and now it seems like I'm getting worse.

Nurse: Why do you think that might be?

Patient: I don't know.

Nurse: You have been given a very difficult disease to manage. And when you don't feel well, it is an even bigger hurdle to jump over.

Patient: It is challenging. But I understand about the food and know what I can and can't eat.

Nurse: (silent)

Patient: Like I said, I did really well for awhile. And the food wasn't too bad, really. But it just got too expensive for me to keep buying.

Nurse: The cost has been a barrier for you.

Patient: It really has. I want to feel good, but I also need to be able to pay my bills. (Ambivalence)

Nurse: That is a difficult choice to make.

Patient: Well, I haven't really had a choice as far as I'm concerned. I need a roof over my family's head and they all need to eat, too.

Nurse: You are very dedicated to your family. You must really love them.

Patient: I do and I don't want them to suffer because I have celiac disease.

Nurse: Often, we feel stuck between a rock and a hard place, but there is often a way out.

Patient: I have thought about going online to see about ordering some food and supplies my wife wants to make me some things. The nutritionist said I might find things cheaper there. (Change talk)

Nurse: That sounds like a great place to start.

Patient: Well, I can't keep living like this. The costs for the emergency room visits are probably costing me more in the long run. And I want to feel good.

Nurse: With your dedication, I trust you will be successful in the management of your celiac disease and keep your family protected at the same time.

Patient: Thank you.

Discussion

The two scenarios provide a completely different approach to the case study presented. The first scenario shows the nurse as authoritative and dictating orders to the patient. The patient was willing to participate in the encounter initially but became passive when the nurse became more aggressive. The nurse was accusatory and blamed the patient for the frequent emergency room visits instead of exploring the true source of his problem. It can be difficult to form a therapeutic relationship when one person acts superior. The patient may have been feeling judged for not properly taking care of himself. If the nurse had taken a step back and elicited additional information from the patient, the outcome could have been more successful.

The second scenario used motivational interviewing tactics. The nurse remained nonjudgmental, explored the patient's perspective, and was able to unearth an entirely different issue. The first scenario showed the nurse assuming the patient was choosing to be "noncompliant." This scenario demonstrated the nurse encouraging the patient to take the journey to explore his personal barriers and possible solutions. The nurse did not recommend any specific steps to take but helped guide the patient in determining what he thought he could realistically do to improve his situation. The nurse used a combination of silence, reflections, and metaphors to encourage patient involvement.

Case Study 2

A patient is considering bariatric surgery. The patient comes to the nurse to discuss this and get more information.

Interaction Without Motivational Interviewing

Nurse: Good morning. What can I help you with today?

Patient: I am interested in bariatric surgery.

Nurse: Okay. Let's go over some things before you make your decision.

Patient: Okay.

Nurse: First let me tell you that this surgery can be a great thing if you need help losing weight. If there is anything you haven't tried, I would try it before doing the surgery.

Patient: I have already tried everything and that is why I'm here.

Nurse: You obviously know the benefits to the surgery. You will be able to lose weight and you will feel much better.

Patient: My main goal is to avoid some problems that will come with being overweight.

Nurse: That will happen, too. There are some risks, such as blood clots, bleeding, obstruction, or infection. After the surgery, you may have problems absorbing certain vitamins or develop anemia. Food may move quickly through your gastrointestinal tract and cause loose stools or diarrhea. And you could have difficulty eating certain foods. When you overeat, you may vomit or have abdominal discomfort. The problem is that most people do not change their way of thinking about eating or their eating patterns.

Patient: I have already changed those habits to prepare for the surgery.

Nurse: So, you should be all set then. I'm glad you came in to talk about this. Good luck with your surgery.

Patient: I was hoping we could talk about the concerns I had about the surgery and if it is the right thing for me.

Nurse: Set up an appointment and we will discuss it further then.

Motivational Interviewing Interaction

Nurse: Good morning. How can I help you today?

Patient: I am interested in bariatric surgery.

Nurse: Tell me what you know about it.

Patient: I have read a lot about it and know what is good and bad about it. I also know that for it to be successful, I need to change my eating habits, but I can't do it. (Resistance)

Nurse: Would you mind sharing with me some of your concerns?

Patient: Well, I know that overeating can cause a lot of problems, and I'm the type of person who eats three large meals a day. I don't have time to snack until bedtime and that is even bigger than it should be.

Nurse: Portion control is difficult for you.

Patient: Exactly. I get so hungry that I just fill my plate and I could have seconds, but I try not to.

Nurse: So, you have made some attempts to decrease your portion sizes but feel you need to improve in that area to be prepared for this surgery.

Patient: Yes, that is true. I just don't think I can do it even though I really want this. I want to lose weight, but I worry that I will not be successful and not sure I can handle the disappointment. (Ambivalence)

Nurse: You are not feeling confident, but there is a drive within you to reach your goal.

Patient: I really want this. Do you have any ideas to help me with my portion sizes? (Change talk)

Nurse: I would be happy to share with you some ideas I have heard from other patients.

Patient: That would be great.

Nurse: I often hear patients tell me how they make up their typical plate and divide it into halves. They spread it out to six smaller meals throughout the day. They often find they cannot eat everything because they have a sensation of being full longer.

Patient: That sounds like something I could do. Thanks for the idea.

Discussion

The scenarios above help to accentuate the benefits of motivational interviewing in brief interactions. The nurse in the first scenario makes assumptions that the patient does not know anything about bariatric surgery. It is important to assess what the patient knows and elicit information to determine what they need to know. When it is determined that information is needed, the nurse should always ask permission to provide education. The nurse did not establish a rapport with the patient. This is important to make the patient feel more comfortable and open up about the issues he or she is facing. When the patient in this scenario states what she needs from the nurse, the nurse dismisses her until another visit. Likely, this patient will not return.

The second scenario is in direct contrast to the first scenario. A rapport was built between the nurse and patient. The patient opened up about a problem she was experiencing that was hindering her from attaining a goal. The nurse asked permission before offering information. The nurse was supportive and encouraging. When motivational interviewing tactics are used, a respectful relationship is formed and the nurse can watch as the patient moves from resistance and blooms into expressing change talk.

Case Study 3

A patient with irritable bowel syndrome comes in for follow-up after being diagnosed 3 months ago.

Interaction Without Motivational Interviewing

Nurse: Good afternoon. How have things been going for you?

Patient: I'm doing better, but I still have a lot of symptoms.

Nurse: Are you taking your medication?

Patient: Yes, I take it just like the doctor told me to.

Nurse: You could be eating too much at a time. Have you been following the diet recommendations?

Patient: Yes. I miss my coffee, but I don't want to make it any worse.

Nurse: What about stress? Do you have anything to be stressed about?

Patient: Doesn't everyone?

Nurse: That's true. Maybe you can exercise or do yoga to help with your stress.

Patient: I do not have time for going to the gym or exercising routinely.

Nurse: It will be important to find ways to manage your stress so that you will have fewer symptoms.

Patient: I am a single mom who works full time and I don't have time for me. Can I get a higher dose of my medicine?

Nurse: You will have to discuss that with the doctor.

Patient: Okay.

Motivational Interviewing Interaction

Nurse: Good afternoon. How have things been going for you?

Patient: Well, my symptoms are definitely improved. But I still have diarrhea and bloating at times.

Nurse: Tell me more.

Patient: It's not every day. But it does interfere with work, and it's hard to get things done at home when I'm not feeling well.

Nurse: Even though your symptoms have improved, they are interfering with your life.

Patient: Yes. I don't have time to be down and out with abdominal pain. I have to work and then I can't be late to pick up the kids at day care. Since I'm a single mom, it's all on my shoulders to make sure they eat and get ready for bed. By the time my day is done, I'm just exhausted as it is and just don't have time to be sick.

Nurse: You have a lot on your plate.

Patient: I guess you could say that.

Nurse: It is difficult to manage all of that and I would think that would produce a lot of stress.

Patient: I'm pretty stressed most of the time.

Nurse: Many patients with irritable bowel syndrome have increased symptoms when they are stressed.

Patient: I think I read that somewhere. I just don't have any options. (Resistance)

Nurse: You must feel hopeless.

Patient: I do sometimes. But I also know that this is my life and I have to deal with the stress of it all. (Ambivalence)

Nurse: There is no escaping life. But there are options. I'm curious how you have managed your stress in the past.

Patient: I used to do meditation. That was before I had my second child. I guess I had a little more free time then.

Nurse: Meditation can be time consuming.

Patient: Actually, I would feel better if I just did it for 15 minutes a day.

Nurse: (silent)

Patient: I might be able to fit that in right before I go to bed at night or maybe when the kids are doing their homework. (Change talk)

Nurse: When you decide to manage your stress, I am confident that you will find a solution that is right for you.

Patient: Thank you.

Discussion

The previous scenarios help to differentiate between effective and ineffective ways to communicate. The first scenario did not result in any behavior change. The patient was resistant, yet the nurse continued to push for stress management. This is when the nurse should "roll with resistance" or ride it out. It is okay for the patient to be resistant. There are reasons why patients resist, and these reasons should be explored to move toward change talk. The nurse portrayed the expert and did not form a partnership with the patient as is helpful when working toward behavior change.

The second scenario is a good example of how motivational interviewing tactics can evoke change talk. Once the nurse established a rapport with the patient, the patient was able to comfortably talk about her personal barriers and reveal that stress was a contributing factor. With the support of the nurse, the patient was able to establish a way to cope with stress in an effort to decrease symptoms of irritable bowel syndrome. The nurse did not take on a directive role and, in fact, encouraged the patient to explore her options and to form her own goals. Promoting behavior change can be very rewarding.

PRACTICE TOOLS (FIGURE 8-2)

1. Be a change agent for your patients. Use motivational interviewing to help patients alter modifiable factors of their gastrointestinal disorder. There are many opportunities to provide support and guidance even in brief interactions, if only we actively listen. It is important not to oversee when a patient is clearly resistant, experiencing ambivalence, or ready to take steps toward change.
2. Motivational interviewing skills can be used in every conversation. There may be conversations about issues that are not directly impacted by a particular behavior that can be changed. Simple behaviors such as hand wash-

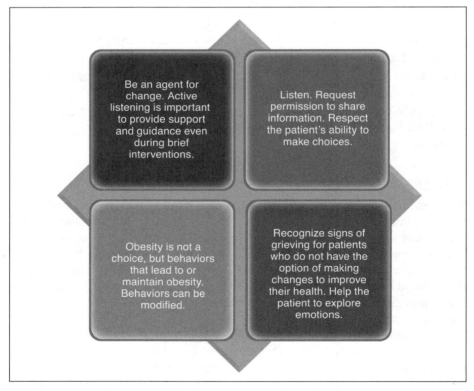

Figure 8-2 Practice Tools

ing can be altered when the patient has the appropriate information. Motivational interviewing encourages the nurse to listen, to request permission to share information, and to accept when the patient makes a choice.

3. Remember that obesity is a major factor that contributes to gastrointestinal and many other disorders. Obesity is not a choice, but there are behaviors that are chosen to be or not to be adopted. This is a struggle that many Americans face. Motivational interviewing can help the patient to explore feelings about his or her weight, evaluate the contributing factors, and determine areas in which he or she can make changes to improve weight. Setting clear, attainable goals is important. By creating a strong, supportive relationship, the nurse can successfully assist the patient to reach a place of comfort and to potentially make changes to improve his or her health.

4. Be aware that some gastrointestinal disorders may not be improved. The patient with cirrhosis of the liver may be facing a liver transplant or death. It is important to recognize signs of grieving that can negatively affect the patient's readiness to change. Sometimes the goal of the patient may be to have a peaceful death. This would require the nurse to promote exploration of the patient's emotions and to allow the patient to make peace with oneself and with loved ones. Motivational interviewing can be a useful tool at this time as well.

5. Use available resources:
   - **American Gastrointestinal Association**
   - American Liver Association
   - **American College of Gastroenterology**
   - **National Digestive Diseases Information Clearinghouse**
   - **National Institute of Diabetes and Digestive and Kidney Diseases**

TAKE-AWAY POINTS

1. Gastrointestinal disorders are common in the United States. Behavior modification needs can range from simple hand washing to changing eating habits, altering the lifestyle in regards to alcohol consumption, caffeine intake, and stress management. The possible uses for motivational interviewing are abundant.

2. More research is needed to prove the effectiveness and explore the possibilities. Motivational interviewing has proven effective in areas of nutrition counseling, weight management, and exercise. All these areas can benefit most people suffering from a gastrointestinal disorder. The goal is to help patients find ways to manage the symptoms of their illness. Research has proven motivational interviewing to be effective in the management of chronic illness.

3. It is sometimes necessary to help the patients think outside of the box. "Creative alternatives are often required to help patients remove obstacles in everyday life that prevent them from achieving their goals" (Mason, 2006, p. 11). Be open to alternative ideas. What the nurse believes to be the best solution may not be best for that particular patient. Appreciate the patient's creativity and encourage exploration of ideas.
4. Often, other issues, such as psychological symptoms, may present barriers to effective communication and behavior change. Motivational interviewing tactics can help the patient address these problems, making it easier to deal with the gastrointestinal disorder.

SUMMARY

In this chapter we explored the impact that gastrointestinal disorders have in the United States. The statistics are astounding and are a driving force, in addition to Healthy People 2010 initiatives, to improve the health of our nation. As with any health disorder, there are challenges to management. As we move toward a focus of self-management, motivational interviewing is an essential tool that nurses should feel comfortable using. This way of communicating with patients can help us to delve deeper into their perspectives and help patients to help themselves. Nurses will always have an opportunity to educate and provide healthcare information. What we need is a more consistent, effective method for communicating with our patients that will successfully lead to better disease management and a higher quality of life. As we see more research being done, motivational interviewing is at the forefront to provide us with an innovative method for promoting behavior change.

REFERENCES

Cash, B. (2005). Advances in functional gastrointestinal disorders. Retrieved June 21, 2009, from cme.medscape.com/viewarticle/515884_ print.

Clark, M., & Slemmons, M. (2008). School programs to reduce the prevalence of obesity in children. *American Journal for Nurse Practitioners, 12*(10), 62–68.

Drossman, D., Talley, N., Leserman, J., Olden, K., & Barreiro, M. (1995). Sexual and physical abuse and gastrointestinal illness: Review and recommendations. *Annals of Internal Medicine, 123*(10), 782–794.

Glovsky, E., & Rose, G. (2007). Motivational interviewing—A unique approach to behavior change counseling. *Today's Dietitian, 9*(5), 50.

Guthrie, E., & Thompson, D. (2002). Abdominal pain and functional gastrointestinal disorders. *British Medical Journal, 325*(7366), 701–703.

Mason, C. (2006). Translating science into patient care: The nurse practitioner's role. Clinical Advisor: A Supplement to the Clinical Advisor, December.

CHAPTER 9

Motivational Interviewing in Genitourinary Health

——— OBJECTIVES ———

After completing this chapter, the reader will be able to

1. Discuss the impact of genitourinary disorders on health in the United States.
2. Identify three challenges in managing complications in genitourinary health.
3. List three benefits of self-management in genitourinary health.
4. Report three areas of genitourinary health that would benefit from the use of motivational interviewing to promote behavior change.
5. Demonstrate appropriate use of reflections when faced with resistance and change talk.

——— KEY TERMS ———

AIDS
Benign prostatic hyperplasia
Chronic kidney disease
End-stage renal disease (ESRD)
HIV
Human papillomavirus
Lower urinary tract symptoms

National Institute of Diabetes and
   Digestive and Kidney Diseases
National Kidney and Urologic
   Diseases Information Clearinghouse
Pelvic inflammatory disease
Urinary tract infection

INTRODUCTION

Genitourinary disorders include disorders of the kidneys, bladder, and prostate; gynecological issues; and sexually transmitted diseases (STDs). Here we examine the prevalence of some of these disorders to evaluate the impact on health in the United States. Many of these disorders can be prevented or improved through changes in behavior. There are many opportunities to use motivational interviewing skills to promote behavior change in these populations.

Between 1999 and 2004 there were approximately 26 million adults with **chronic kidney disease**. By 2006 there were over ½ million people being treated for **end-stage renal disease (ESRD)**. In that same year almost 90,000 people died from ESRD. The cost of treatment approached $34 billion. The most recent data in 2006 revealed that 18,052 kidney transplants were performed. In October 2008 about 80,000 people were awaiting transplants for kidneys alone or kidney with pancreas.

The effect of ESRD can be devastating. The most common causes for ESRD are diabetes and hypertension. By controlling these two diseases, the rate of ESRD could decrease tremendously. Many cases of diabetes and hypertension can either be prevented or controlled, mainly by diet, exercise, and weight management (see http://kidney.niddk.nih.gov/kudiseases/pubs/kustats/index.htm).

Urinary tract infections are quite common but are preventable in some cases. In 2006 there were about 479,000 inpatient hospital stays due to urinary tract infections. In 2000 there were about 19 million outpatient visits for urinary tract infections. The estimated cost for treatment in 2000 was $3.5 billion. We often do not consider urinary tract infections to be serious because they are easily treated in most cases. Despite the ease of treatment, it is a common occurrence and has a significant financial impact on our country. Helping patients to recognize common causes and behaviors that could help prevent the occurrence can be accomplished through the use of motivational interviewing (see http://kidney.niddk.nih.gov/kudiseases/pubs/kustats/index.htm).

Enuresis, or urinary incontinence, not only affects children but also adults. In fact, this condition can be more devastating to the adult population. The following statistical information is related to the adult population. Between 1999 and 2000, 38% of women and 17% of men aged 60 years old and over were afflicted by this condition. There were almost 50,000 hospital stays and about 4.5 million outpatient visits for adults aged 20 years and over. The total cost in 2000 for inpatient and outpatient treatment was $463.1 million. This condition is not life threatening and does not have serious consequences, but it still has an impact financially and on the emotional status of the patients afflicted. Through the use of motivational interviewing, tactics to help cope with or improve the condition can be brought to light (see http://kidney.niddk.nih.gov/kudiseases/pubs/kustats/index.htm).

Men can have their own set of problems, such as prostate enlargement and erectile dysfunction. An enlarged prostate can lead to **benign prostatic hyperplasia** or **lower urinary tract symptoms**. In 2000, 6.5 million men, ages 50–79, were at the stage of discussing treatment options. A little over 12 million doctor visits occurred in 2000 for men aged 20 and older. Direct costs that same year for enlarged prostate issues totaled $1.1 billion. Erectile dysfunction can happen at any age, but the incidence increases with age and can be a secondary problem to a primary diagnosis, such as diabetes. In 2000, 6.2% of men aged 20 and older were reported to have been afflicted. This can be a difficult topic for men to discuss, and the use of motivational interviewing provides the respect and support the patient needs to feel comfortable talking with the provider (see http://kidney.niddk.nih.gov/kudiseases/pubs/kustats/index.htm).

There are many issues experienced by women alone. Endometriosis, ovarian cysts, issues with fertility, and menopause are only a few topics that come up when working in women's health. The Robert Wood Johnson University Hospital reported that endometriosis occurs in about 10–20% of females of child-bearing age. Endometriosis is one of the major causes of infertility in women. **Pelvic inflammatory disease** is a common complication of STDs and can also lead to infertility. More than 1 million women experience pelvic inflammatory disease per year. Chlamydia is the most frequently reported STD, with 75% who are asymptomatic and may not seek out health care for that reason. Given these statistics there is an incredible need to focus on this area to improve the health of our female population. Ovarian cancer is most likely to cause death than any other cancer of the reproductive system. It is also the sixth most common form of cancer in the female population (see http://www.rwjuh.edu/health_information/adult_gyneonc_stats.html).

STDs are significantly challenging yet entirely preventable. The Centers for Disease Control and Prevention (CDC) publishes updated statistical data on STDs each year. As previously stated, chlamydia is the most commonly reported STD. There were 1,108,374 cases of chlamydia reported in 2007. More women than men were diagnosed, but there has been an increase in the number of males diagnosed since initiating urine testing for chlamydia. There were 355,991 cases of gonorrhea reported in 2007, which was not significantly changed from the previous year. Again, more cases were reported in women than in men. Despite the surgeon general's goal to eradicate syphilis, there were 11,466 cases reported in 2007. There were more men than women diagnosed. Cases of congenital syphilis are also on the rise, with 430 cases reported in 2007 (CDC, 2008). Motivational interviewing can have a significant impact on promoting behavior change that can lead to a decrease in the incidence of STDs.

HIV is an STD that deserves special attention because of the risk of progressing to **AIDS** and ultimately death. The toll it has taken on our population is unfortunate because it can be prevented. By the end of 2007 there were 337,590 total cases of HIV reported to the CDC; of these, 75% were male and 657 cases were in children. There were 1,030,832 persons with AIDS at that time. Seventy-four percent were males, and 87 cases were in children. AIDS caused about 2 million deaths in 2007. It is reported that about 5,500 people die each day from AIDS. These astounding statistics reinforce the need for prevention and behavior change, which can be accomplished through the use of motivational interviewing tactics (CDC, 2009; see http://www.usaid.gov/our_work/global_health/aids/News/aidsfaq.html).

Healthy People 2010 designated focus areas that are related to genitourinary health. Chronic kidney disease is one of these focus areas. Chronic kidney disease can be caused by other diagnoses such as diabetes. It can lead to ESRD, which is a devastating disease that leaves little treatment options. There is a drive to decrease STDs, with HIV being a focus area of its own because of its impact on our population. Immunization as a form of prevention is also important because there is a vaccination to prevent the **human papillomavirus**, which is targeted at young women to decrease the risk of cervical cancer. In 2003–2004 the CDC reported a 26.8% prevalence rate in noninstitutionalized women. A portion of those were preventable with the use of Gardisil for immunization. Hopefully, positive data will be reported over the next several years due to the initiation of Gardisil (CDC, 2009; see http://www.healthypeople.gov/About/hpfact.htm).

CHALLENGES IN GENITOURINARY HEALTH

There are many challenges in caring for patients with problems affecting their genitourinary health. Consider the patient with ESRD. This is a person whose life is only prolonged with treatment, and the quality of life is significantly decreased. Now consider trying to help promote behavior change with this patient. A number of responses, such as the following, put up roadblocks:

- "I don't want dialysis. I want to enjoy my last days."
- "What does it matter if I drink? I'm going to die anyway."
- "It doesn't matter what I eat. My kidneys are already damaged. I can't do any more damage to them."
- "I have so many other health problems to deal with that caused my kidneys to fail. I have to focus on other things right now."

Many patients are dealing with grief and end-of-life issues; what the nurse wants to focus on to improve patients' health is not an issue for them. This is where the spirit of motivational interviewing is helpful. The nurse's role is not to decide what is best for the patient but to in fact help the patient decide what he or she wants and how to get there. This may mean the patient will exhibit negative behaviors and the nurse must be accepting and nonjudgmental. Change for patients may be to stop doing everything they can to improve their health and to enjoy what life they have left. Quality of death is just as important as quality of life.

Chronic genitourinary problems can be difficult for the patient to manage, yet he or she is the one responsible to make choices each day related to his or her illness. "Accordingly, even a patient's not managing a chronic illness reflects a decision about management" (Thomas-Hawkins & Zazworsky, 2005, p. 41). Each person has his or her own understanding and methods of managing. There is no set way to approach every patient. That is why it is important to get to know the patient and build a rapport. It is difficult to "let go" and let the patient guide the way. We need to be able to sit back, listen attentively, and, when possible, provide gentle guidance in the direction they want to go.

Another challenge in this arena is that some of the topics are difficult for both patients and nurses to discuss. Nurses must overcome their discomforts to make it a more open environment to invite the patient to talk about uncomfortable issues. Sexual health is natural and needs to be treated as such. Topics such as erectile dysfunction, infertility, and STDs need to be handled openly and without judgment. Many people feel shame when they are diagnosed with an STD. The nurse should help to empower the patient to have the self-confidence that is needed to make positive choices in regard to their sexual health.

Yet another challenge is discussion of safe sexual practice, which should be a common topic for patient encounters. We have not been as effective in this area, thus the statistical data discussed previously that reveal a significant problem facing the United States population. Knowing when to discuss and the best way to approach this topic is difficult.

Having time limits on patient encounters also proves challenging. We struggle to find enough time in the day to get the basics done. It is overwhelming to think of adding one more task or learning a new way of doing things. But as the world around us changes, we must change too. Motivational interviewing is one method of helping to ease the weight of the changes. Once this method is mastered, you will find it does not take a lot of time to make a difference.

BENEFITS OF SELF-MANAGEMENT

Self-management is not only beneficial but necessary. Motivational interviewing is one way to help promote self-management by encouraging self-efficacy. Many trials have been done in relation to self-management of chronic diseases, such as diabetes and asthma. Reviewers of these studies found it difficult to get an accurate picture of the effectiveness of evaluating self-management due to the diversity of methods used (Thomas-Hawkins & Zazworsky, 2005). What we do know is that care providers spend minimal time with patients and that patients are the ones who carry out the tasks each day. Our job is to help them do that with as much knowledge and self-confidence as possible to be effective. Motivational interviewing offers us the tools to accomplish this. "Motivational Interviewing has been successfully used in the treatment of addictions and could be applied to many areas of health care in both hospital and community settings. Motivational interviewing can easily find a place in health promotion and treating persons dealing with the consequences of chronic illness such as diabetes, heart disease and chronic kidney disease" (Ossman, 2004).

In an article about self-management in chronic kidney disease, Thomas-Hawkins and Zazworsky (2005) reviewed the need to assess the patient's understanding and readiness to change and help promote self-efficacy. They also spoke of the need for support. In one study "the nursing intervention involved teaching patients stress-management techniques, helping them to identify problem areas in their self-management, and allowing them to express their feelings" (Thomas-Hawkins & Zazworsky, 2005, p. 46). By doing so they were able to see improvement in the patient's self-confidence in self-management (Thomas-Hawkins & Zazworsky, 2005). It is difficult to take steps toward change alone. Nurse support can be crucial to promoting behavior change.

Motivating a patient is not always simple. Karalis and Wiesen (2007) reviewed how to incorporate motivational interviewing into the care of the renal patient. They emphasized the ease of motivating patients and provided ways to motivate patients that goes with the spirit of motivational interviewing (Figure 9-1). Not only are the tools helpful for working with patients with ESRD, but they can be transferred to working with patients with other chronic illnesses. The authors suggested that motivation can come from offering support and encouragement and working with the patient rather than telling the patient what to do (Karalis & Wiesen, 2007).

As with many illnesses, there is a crossover effect on the outcomes of other diseases. While on dialysis there is an increased risk for cerebrovascular disease. Maintaining healthy behaviors even at this stage of a disease can significantly decrease the risk for other complications. If we can help improve any negative health behaviors, we can potentially decrease the risk of complications that can lead to a decreased quality of life or even death (Sozio et al., 2009).

The use of motivational interviewing in the area of sexual health or STDs has been found to be effective. One study recognized that there were not enough studies to prove effectiveness and performed a study using motivational interviewing in the care of people living with HIV. Staff received training in motivational interviewing and used it with their clients. The nurses felt more confident about their role and the use of motivational interviewing. They learned to recognize that not everyone wants to change. The nurses also learned the positive impact of helping patients to look at themselves and their life and to evaluate the positive and negative aspects of changing negative behavior (Byrne, Watson, Butler, & Accoroni, 2006).

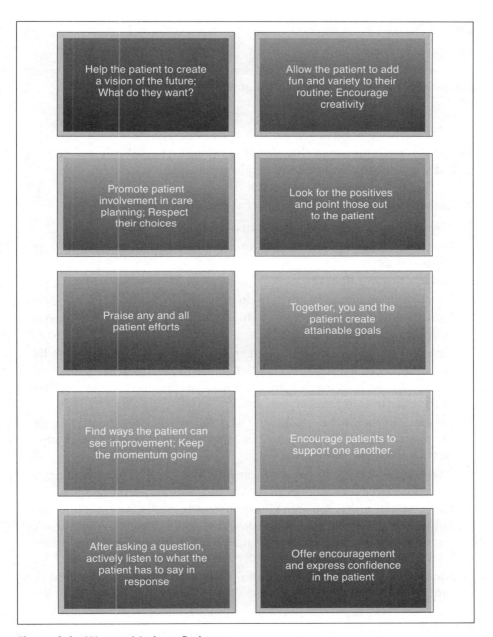

Figure 9-1   Ways to Motivate Patients

Source: Adapted from Karalis, M. & Wiesen, K., 2007.

CASE STUDIES

The following case studies represent interactions with and without the use of motivational interviewing tactics. A discussion follows each case study regarding the effective and ineffective techniques used.

Case Study 1

The patient has a history of chronic kidney disease. His diabetes is poorly controlled and is the likely cause for the kidney damage.

Interaction Without Motivational Interviewing

Nurse: Good morning. How are you doing today?

Patient: I'm okay, I guess. The doctor just told me that I might have to go on dialysis soon.

Nurse: I'm sorry to hear that.

Patient: I don't think I'm going to do it.

Nurse: I don't understand. I thought you would want to do it to extend your life.

Patient: I'm not looking for a longer life. I want what I have left to be good. And I can tell you that being on dialysis would not be a good life.

Nurse: Well, without dialysis you won't have any life, and I would urge you to consider it. Your family needs you.

Patient: They need me as someone who can be there for them, support them, and take care of them, not the other way around. They aren't supposed to take care of me.

Nurse: Obviously, you need some time to think about it. We are going to have you placed on a transplant list...

Patient: (interrupts) You aren't listening to me. I've lived a good life. I do not want a transplant. I already know that could take years and I don't want dialysis. I want to enjoy what time I have with my family and when it's my time to go, I will go peacefully. I don't want to be saved.

Nurse: Okay. I will let your doctor know what you have told me and I'm sure he will give you a call.

Motivational Interviewing Interaction

Nurse: Good morning. How are you?

Patient: I'm okay. I've been having a hard time since the doctor told me I may need to start dialysis soon.

Nurse: Tell me about that.

Patient: Well, I knew the day would come. I just didn't know how it would feel to hear it. I thought I knew exactly what I would want to do when this happened, but I don't know.

Nurse: It's a difficult time and a big decision to make.

Patient: Some people think there's no decision, you just do it. But I don't really want to.

Nurse: (silent)

Patient: I have thought about it and thought about it. Dialysis just isn't for me. I want to enjoy my life. For me, it's about quality, not quantity. (Resistance)

Nurse: Even if you have less time here, you want to be able to enjoy it. You feel you won't be able to enjoy it on dialysis.

Patient: No, I wouldn't. I see how exhausted people are after dialysis. My father was on dialysis and it was horrible to see him living that way. I don't want to spend my last days sleeping. What kind of life is that?

Nurse: I'm curious about what you feel the pros and the cons are in this situation.

Patient: Well, I think the pros are that by not doing dialysis, I have more immediate time to spend with my family. I know that dialysis can be time consuming. I also know that it would be good to make peace with myself and my family while I'm still feeling up to it.

Nurse: (silent)

Patient: The negatives would obviously be that I will die sooner. I have a hard time imagining that I am dying. I wish there was something other than dialysis that would keep me going longer. I guess another negative would be my family not really understanding or supporting my decision. I know they would want me to do the dialysis.

Nurse: There is a conflict between what you want and what your family wants.

Patient: Yes. That's what I really need the help with. I need to know how to help my family accept my decision.

Nurse: What are your thoughts about how that conversation might go?

Patient: My son will be the only one to understand and might be okay with it. I know my wife and daughter will cry and beg me to try it.

Nurse: Whereas your son would be most likely to walk down that path with you, you are afraid your wife and daughter will try to hold you back.

Patient: I know they will. They are very emotional and I can't stand to see them cry. Maybe I should tell my son first so he can help me talk with them.

Nurse: That might be a good idea. You can enlist his support.

Patient: Just having someone there with me will make a huge difference. And if they have questions, can they talk with you?

Nurse: Absolutely. If there is anything I can do to help get you through this, I would be happy to help. You have obviously put a lot of thought into this and I support what choices you make.

Discussion

The previous two scenarios have very different outcomes. Being faced with something as life changing as ESRD can be devastating. The nurse can tell the patient what is needed to improve the situation from a health perspective or walk beside the patient and offer support and encouragement as the patient makes choices.

The first scenario does not use motivational interviewing tactics and results in the nurse being more forceful about the issue of dialysis. The nurse assumes that all patients want to extend their life. Placing our assumptions on a patient will result in resistance and a rapid end to the conversation. The patient feels unheard, and the nurse is frustrated.

The second scenario demonstrates the use of motivational interviewing and results in a partnership to accomplishing the patient's goal. The patient may be resistant to treatment and feels comfortable discussing with the nurse because they had built a rapport. There was not a particular behavior they worked to change. Instead, the patient and nurse worked together to come up with a way of dealing with an issue brought about by the patient's diagnosis. At the end of the second scenario there is a sense that the patient and nurse worked together as a team. The nurse did not pass judgment but explored the patient's perspective to better understand the choice he had made.

Case Study 2

The patient comes in for STD testing. She is concerned she is at risk due to a previous unprotected contact with a partner who has an STD.

Interaction Without Motivational Interviewing

Nurse: Good morning. I see you are here today for testing.

Patient: Yes.

Nurse: I have looked over your risk evaluation and can see that it would be appropriate to test you. Before we get started, we should talk about ways to prevent STDs from occurring.

Patient: Well, I have used condoms at times.

Nurse: Condoms should be used every time there is a sexual encounter. There is no room to take risks. Do you understand how serious it would be to have HIV or AIDS?

Patient: I doubt I have any STD; I just got worried there could be a chance. And I do take birth control.

Nurse: Birth control can only help prevent pregnancy and will not offer any protection against STDs.

Patient: Well, I figure some protection is better than no protection.

Nurse: Unfortunately, it isn't really helpful if you don't practice safer sex to avoid pregnancy and STDs.

Patient: Okay.

Nurse: Now let's talk about how you can prevent STDs.

Motivational Interviewing Interaction

Nurse: Good morning. How can I help you today?

Patient: I thought I should come in and get tested for any STDs.

Nurse: We are more than happy to help with that. Usually, we go through the risk factors to determine your level of risk, do the testing, and discuss ways to protect yourself in the future.

Patient: Oh, I don't think I need to worry about the future. I now have one boyfriend, so I don't think I have any more risks. (Resistance)

Nurse: You feel that being in a monogamous relationship protects you.

Patient: Of course it does. If we are only having sex with each other, then there is no problem.

Nurse: I'm curious if your boyfriend is being tested or plans to be tested, also.

Patient: He doesn't want to and I didn't push it. He has only been with a few girls lately and his wild days were quite awhile ago.

Nurse: It is easy to think we are the only one when we are in a relationship and do not want to think about past relationships. In fact, those past relationships also had past relationships, and it can be difficult to know what could have been passed from one person to another.

Patient: I guess you are right. He did have one girlfriend that was pretty promiscuous. Who knows how many sexual contacts she has had.

Nurse: It is something we often do not consider when we are looking at our risk factors.

Patient: I want to trust that he has nothing he could give me, but I just don't know, now that I think about it. (Ambivalence)

Nurse: You want to go into this relationship without worry, but without knowing if he has an STD may cause concern.

Patient: Absolutely. I want to do the testing today and would be happy to hear how I can protect myself.

Nurse: I would be happy to help with that. Tell me how you might handle the situation with your current boyfriend.

Patient: I am going to have to talk to him. I will only have sex if he wears a condom and he needs to know how important it is to me for him to be tested also. (Change talk)

Nurse: How do you plan to approach this with your boyfriend?

Patient: I am just going to have to ask him again and tell him that I need to know if we are ever going to have sex without a condom.

Nurse: Being straightforward is a good idea. If he has any questions or if we can help him here with the testing, have him call me.

Discussion

The previous two scenarios compare how a nonmotivational interviewing and a motivational interviewing interaction are different. The first scenario leaves the patient feeling judged, and there is obvious resistance. The nurse is authoritative and this is an obvious barrier to effective communication. The nurse clearly wanted to discuss methods of prevention, but the patient had a knowledge gap, and this should have been addressed. When there is a lack of knowledge, the nurse should ask permission to share information to increase the knowledge. Once the patient has a better understanding, the nurse can then proceed to topics the patient is interested in discussing.

The second scenario used respectful communication as encouraged by motivational interviewing. The nurse asked open-ended questions and offered reflections to demonstrate she was listening. There was a rapport between the nurse and patient that promoted open communication. The nurse was able to elicit the information regarding the reasons the patient wanted testing and a gap in knowledge. The patient accepted the information, and this helped her to make informed decisions about how to proceed. This scenario was clearly more successful in the development of the nurse–patient relationship and the outcome of the interaction.

Case Study 3

The patient is in for a routine physical. He has a history of type 2 diabetes and hypertension. Recently, he has been suffering from erectile dysfunction.

Interaction Without Motivational Interviewing

Nurse: Good morning. How have you been?

Patient: I've been pretty good.

Nurse: I see you are here for your physical. Do you have any concerns?

Patient: Well, I think the only thing that has been a problem is that. . . . Well, I'm having a problem getting an erection.

Nurse: Oh, you are having what is called erectile dysfunction.

Patient: Yeah, I guess that's what I've heard it called on the commercials.

Nurse: Let me ask, how is your diabetes control?

Patient: Well, it isn't great. I've been having a hard time getting my numbers under control.

Nurse: You need to have better control of the diabetes; otherwise you will have problems like these.

Patient: I know and I've been trying.

Nurse: Make sure you follow-up with your diabetes doctor. You can get undressed now and the doctor will be in soon to examine you.

Motivational Interviewing Interaction

Nurse: Good morning. How are you doing?

Patient: I'm okay, I guess.

Nurse: I see you are here for a physical. Do you have any concerns you would like to discuss?

Patient: Well, I do have one thing that has been bothering me.

Nurse: (silent)

Patient: I was hoping to talk to the doctor about getting some Viagra. I am having that kind of a problem.

Nurse: Many people suffer from erectile dysfunction, especially people with diabetes. Do you mind my asking how long this has been a problem?

Patient: It started about 6 months ago and is worse now.

Nurse: It has been a problem, but now you would like to do something about it.

Patient: Yes. I want to know why this is happening to me. The diabetes doctor said my diabetes is not so good lately. Do you think that has anything to do with it? (Change talk)

Nurse: There is a connection. When diabetes is poorly controlled, it can lead to problems such as this. What are your thoughts?

Patient: Well, I remember learning something about that being a possible problem. I guess I just didn't think this would ever happen to me.

Nurse: What do you feel you can do to help the situation?

Patient: I want to get the medication from the doctor, but I also need to work on my diabetes control.

Nurse: On one hand, you want immediate relief, but at the same time, you are looking to improve the situation by improving your diabetes control.

Patient: That is right.

Nurse: That sounds like a great place to start. You can discuss the medication with the doctor and I would be happy to help you with the diabetes.

Patient: Thank you. I know what I need to do. I just need to do it.

Discussion

The previous two scenarios demonstrate two very different approaches to the same encounter. In the first scenario the patient comes to the nurse with a concern about erectile dysfunction, and the nurse turned it into a conversation about the patient's diabetes control. The patient was not heard, and the focus of the conversation was nurse directed. The nurse was clearly not listening to what was on the patient's mind. The nurse also completely disregarded the patient's concern. This patient may not feel comfortable approaching the topic with the physician after such disregard from the nurse.

The second scenario revealed a more effective encounter. The patient did not show resistance and was clearly ready to make changes if it would improve his situation. The nurse listened to what the patient said and let the patient guide the conversation. The nurse was able to help the patient see the connection between his current issue and the management of his diabetes. Because he wanted to change his current situation, he was willing, in fact eager, to make some changes in his diabetes. Not every encounter is met with resistance. Some patients have already gone through the thought process and come to you ready to make changes.

PRACTICE TOOLS (FIGURE 9-2)

1. Walk with your patients. Let them decide the pace and direction of the encounter. At times the patient may be happy with where they are or may not be ready for change. When we encounter resistance, it is often something we have said that pushes them away. "Your desire to encourage change can lead you into a persuasion-resistance trap: The harder you persuade, the more the patient resists" (Rollnick, Miller, & Butler, 2008, p. 148).

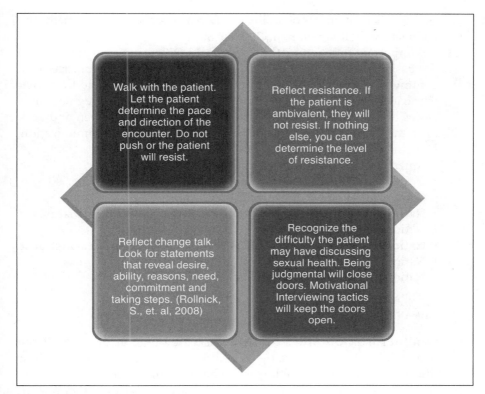

Figure 9-2 Practice Tools

2. People with ESRD and AIDS are dealing with a terminal illness and may not be interested in change. It will be important to "roll with resistance" and even "reflect resistance." "Because people who feel ambivalent have both sides of the argument within them, they will often back away from resistance when you reflect it nonjudgmentally. Even if they do not, you will get a clearer picture of the patient's resistance" (Rollnick et al., 2008, p. 79).
3. Some patients come to the encounter looking to change behaviors. Using the motivational interviewing guiding style, the nurse will follow the patient's lead. The nurse may feel there are more important areas to focus on, but when the patient comes with motivation to change it is an opportunity that cannot be passed up. Instead of having to evoke the change talk, it is right there before you and you should "reflect change talk." "In other words, what you particularly want to reflect, when you hear it, is

change talk (statements of desire, ability, reasons, need, commitment, and taking steps)" (Rollnick et al., 2008, p. 80).
4. It is important to recognize the discomfort a patient may experience when discussing sexual health. Remain nonjudgmental and encourage open communication. Patients are most likely to open up and address their true concerns when they feel comfortable with the nurse. Judgment only closes doors. Motivational interviewing tactics help to open and keep open the doors that are common barriers to therapeutic communication.
5. Use available resources:
   • American College of Obstetricians and Gynecologists
   • American Urological Association
   • Centers for Disease Control and Prevention
   • **National Institute of Diabetes and Digestive and Kidney Diseases**
   • National Institutes of Health
   • **National Kidney and Urologic Diseases Information Clearinghouse**
   • National Kidney Disease Education Program
   • National Kidney Foundation

TAKE-AWAY POINTS

1. Genitourinary disorders constitute a wide range of disorders from women's health, men's health, STDs, to renal disorders. Some of these disorders have a significant impact on health in the United States. We lose thousands of people each day to diseases such as ESRD and AIDS. A focus on prevention could have a positive effect on the statistics surrounding these diseases. Motivational interviewing has been found to be effective in the areas of ESRD and AIDS. Motivational interviewing tactics can be beneficial in numerous other areas as well.
2. Many issues that come up in an encounter are a product of another problem or disease. The patient may benefit from addressing the source of the problem or may want to focus only on his or her present concern. Recognizing when a patient is ready to focus on the source of the problem is important. It is easy to fall into the trap of the "righting reflex" and want to force the direction the interaction will take. Increasing self-awareness will help avoid this trap.
3. Healthy People 2010 maintains a strong focus on prevention and control of HIV, AIDS, and other STDs. Negative health behaviors are large contributors to these problems. Motivational interviewing has been found to be effective in promoting behavior change in these areas. Proper utilization of the tools can help to decrease the prevalence of these diseases and lead us to a healthier nation, the ultimate goal of Healthy People 2010.

4. It is okay for people to not make a change. We need to appreciate their right to resist change. It is challenging to see a patient be noncompliant, not adhere to treatment recommendations, and choose to simply accept where they are. Although it is difficult to understand a person's desire to not treat an illness, we need to support that person's choices. On the other side, some patients do not need us to elucidate the importance of change. They can come to us ready to change, and our role is to simply walk with them and support them in finding a way to accomplish their goals.

SUMMARY

Throughout this chapter we have looked at different ways that motivational interviewing can be used in managing genitourinary health. We can use the tools to promote behavior change in areas of prevention, self-management, and treatment of diseases. With STDs and HIV/AIDS having an incredible impact on our population's health, it is not surprising that Healthy People 2010 focuses on these areas. Chronic kidney disease and ESRD also have a place in the Healthy People 2010 focus areas. As we strive to attain the goals set for our nation, we can take comfort in knowing we are armed with tools from motivational interviewing that, when used properly, can help us to establish a healthier nation. As we move toward Healthy People 2020, we can begin a new decade of goals with confidence and self-assurance.

REFERENCES

Byrne, A., Watson, R., Butler, C., & Accoroni, A. (2006). Increasing the confidence of nursing staff to address the sexual health needs of people living with HIV: The use of motivational interviewing. *AIDS Care, 18*(5), 501–504.

Centers for Disease Control and Prevention [CDC]. (2008). *Sexually transmitted disease surveillance, 2007.* Atlanta, GA: U.S. Department of Health and Human Services.

Centers for Disease Control and Prevention [CDC]. (2009). *HIV/AIDS surveillance report, 2007* (volume 19). Atlanta, GA: U.S. Department of Health and Human Services.

Karalis, M., & Wiesen, K. (2007). Motivational interviewing. *Nephrology Nursing Journal, 34*(3), 336–338.

Ossman, S. (2004). Motivational interviewing: A process to encourage behavioral change. *Nephrology Nursing Journal,* May-June. Retrieved September 28, 2008, from http://findarticles.com/p/articles/mi_m0ICF/is_3_31/ai_n17207258/print?tag=artBody:col1.

Rollnick, S., Miller, W., & Butler, C. (2008). *Motivational interviewing in health care: Helping patients change behavior.* New York: The Guilford Press.

Sozio, S., Armstrong, P., Coresh, J., Jaar, B., Fink, N., Plantinga, L., Powe, N., & Parekh, R. (2009). Cerebrovascular disease incidence, characteristics, and outcomes in patients initiating dialysis: The choices for healthy outcomes in caring for ESRD (CHOICE) study. *American Journal of Kidney Diseases, 54*(3), 468–477.

Thomas-Hawkins, C., & Zazworsky, D. (2005). Self-management of chronic kidney disease. *American Journal of Nursing, 105*(10), 40–48.

CHAPTER 10

Motivational Interviewing in Neurological Disorders

INTRODUCTION

Neurological disorders can be devastating to patients and their families. The impact these disorders have on our nation is astounding. The disorders range from Alzheimer's and Parkinson's disease, **multiple sclerosis (MS)**, headaches, to pain. There are numerous other disorders, but because of the scope of this text we focus on some of the most prominent disorders. Some of these disorders are thought to affect our elderly population but, as with any other disease, can impact the lives of younger adults and children.

Parkinson's disease is primarily a movement disorder that can cause difficulty with tremors, gait, mobility, and speech and often triggers the onset of depression.

It is thought that 10 of every 1,000 elderly Americans suffer with this affliction. Typically, this disorder affects people over the age of 65. There are approximately 60,000 people diagnosed each year in the United States. There are about 1.5 million Americans with Parkinson's disease, and 15% of those are diagnosed before the age of 50. The **American Parkinson Disease Association** has the National Young Onset Center for those diagnosed younger than 50 years of age. They recognize the additional issues that arise in this younger population. These statistics were gathered for publication in 2007. Clearly, there is a need to address the many physical and psychosocial issues that can come with such a devastating disease (see http://www.parkinson.org/Page.aspx?pid=225 and http://www.sciencedaily.com/releases/2007/01/070129172536.htm).

Amyotrophic lateral sclerosis (ALS), once referred to as "Lou Gehrig's disease," is another neuromuscular disorder. This progressive, degenerative disorder leaves the patient with areas of paralysis and a life expectancy of approximately 3–5 years after diagnosis. There are on average 30,000 people with this disorder, and 5,600 are diagnosed each year. The typical population afflicted includes those from ages 40 to 70 years. In the younger population more men than women are diagnosed, but the male-to-female ratio is more equal in the older populations. Unfortunately, because of the progression of this disease and the lack of a cure, the focus of treatment is symptom management. Depression is common in this disorder as a result of difficulty communicating as the disease progresses, lack of independence, and feelings of isolation (Farley, 2004).

Approximately 3 million Americans are diagnosed with epilepsy and seizures. This includes children and adults. The cost of managing these disorders is about $15.5 billion. Two hundred thousand people are diagnosed with a seizure each year, with 75,000 to 100,000 younger than 5 years of age and being fever related. There are about 200,000 people diagnosed with epilepsy each year. Those at greatest risk are less than 2 or greater than 65 years of age. Forty-five thousand of these cases are children younger than age 15. Only 70% of those people with epilepsy can expect to go into "remission" or be seizure free with the use of medication for 5 or more years (see http://www.epilepsyfoundation.org/about/statistics.cfm).

Alzheimer's disease is the sixth leading cause of death in our country. There has been an increased awareness due to publicity that this disease has received. It is estimated that 5.3 million people suffer from Alzheimer's disease, with someone being diagnosed every 70 seconds. This is astounding when put into this perspective. One hundred forty-eight billion dollars are spent each year due to this devastating disease. Because of the cognitive decline these patients face, they require someone to provide care 24 hours a day. Approximately 9.9 million people are providing care for these patients without pay. They may be family or friends of those afflicted. In 2008 caregivers provided 8.5 billion hours of unpaid care, translating into $94 billion of additional money that could have been spent on managing this disease. Although this disease primarily affects the older population, it is not a normal part of aging. From another perspective, Alzheimer's disease is predicted to affect an estimated 7.7 million people by 2030. With these present statistics and prediction for the future, it is only reasonable to expect these patients to need healthcare providers that can support the caregivers (Alzheimer's Association, 2009).

Muscular dystrophy is another neuromuscular disorder that is progressive and degenerative. It is considered a genetic disorder that has various forms. Duchenne muscular dystrophy primarily affects children between ages 3 and 5 and progresses rapidly. Becker muscular dystrophy is similar but has a slower progression. Facioscapulohumeral muscular dystrophy is diagnosed in the teenage years, progresses slowly, but ultimate prognosis varies from mild symptoms to disabling. Myotonic muscular dystrophy affects adults and has comorbidities of cataracts and cardiac and endocrine disorders.

There are a number of other forms of muscular dystrophy. Specific statistics are not readily available. From the information that is available, we can conclude that this is yet another devastating neurological disorder that deserves attention. There is no cure, and patients and their families look to us for guidance and support. Daily choices must be made in the management of these disorders. Motivational interviewing can certainly help those who must make the choices that impact the care of the patient, who may or may not be able to care for themselves (see http://www.ninds.nih.gov/disorders/md/md.htm).

According to the National Institute of Neurological Disorders and Stroke, there are about 250,000 to 350,000 people living with MS in the United States. An estimated 200 people are diagnosed with MS each week. It is difficult to diagnose, but in retrospect most people have initial symptoms between the ages of 20 and 40. As with many neurological disorders, this is a progressive illness, but patients typically have a normal life expectancy. Women are more likely to be afflicted. Young children and older adults have been diagnosed, but this is a rare occurrence. The cost of managing MS is not clear but is thought to be in the billions of dollars. There are many symptoms of MS, such as fatigue, pain, muscle weakness, genitourinary dysfunction, and changes in speech, vision, cognition, and depression. Many of these areas are topics of conversations that could benefit from the use of motivational interviewing (see http://www.ninds.nih.gov/disorders/multiple_sclerosis/detail_multiple_sclerosis.htm).

A number of brain and spinal cord injuries occur each year. These types of injuries contribute to problems with voluntary and involuntary muscle movement, cognition, sensation, communication, and behavior. Depending on the patient's abilities, health promotion efforts are focused on the patient and/or caregiver. Most of the 1.4 million brain injury documented cases are mild or diagnosed as concussions. It is estimated that 11,000 people sustain a spinal cord injury each year. The most common causes include motor vehicle accidents and sports-related injuries. According to the Centers for Disease Control and Prevention, at least $9.7 billion are spent each year on the care of patients with spinal cord injuries. Approximately 200,000 people in the United States live with disability of some form as a result of a spinal cord injury. Most of these cases are between the ages of 15 and 29. Some of these injuries can leave the patient paralyzed or mentally incapacitated (see http://www.cdc.gov/TraumaticBrainInjury/physicians_tool_kit.html and http://www.cdc.gov/ncipc/factsheets/scifacts.htm).

Autism spectrum disorders (ASDs) are a group of disorders that have become a topic of interest over the past few years. Because the spectrum of disorders ranges from autistic disorder, to higher functioning form of Asperger's syndrome, it is difficult to determine how many people are truly afflicted. **Pervasive developmental disorders** are part of this spectrum and can be further broken down into subcategories of Rett's syndrome and childhood disintegrative disorder. The earliest time of diagnosis is typically around 18 months. In 2007 data released estimated about 1 in 150 children aged 8 years had some form of ASD. Behavior management is important in managing this spectrum of disorders but is only one aspect of treatment. Motivational interviewing can significantly help those who are higher functioning or the parents of the lower functioning children. Applied behavioral analysis is a form of treatment that is commonly used for ASDs. This is very time consuming for the child and parent, with a recommended 40 hours per week of dedicated time. There is a significant impact on the child and entire family of those who have an ASD. Many of these children need structure and strict regimens that are difficult to adhere to due to the time factor. Motivational interviewing has been found to be effective in improving treatment adherence in a number of areas. Although it has not been studied in this particular area, it could prove to be beneficial (see http://.cdc.gov/ncbddd/autism/overview.htm and http://autism.about.com/od/alllaboutaba/a/abaoverview_2.htm).

As we work toward attaining the goals of Healthy People 2010, some focus areas are pertinent to the neurological disorders. The sixth focus area listed is for disability and secondary conditions. Neurological disorders are a significant cause for disability and require a variety of interventions to improve the health of those afflicted.

From a different perspective, there has been a lot of debate over the safety of certain immunizations, which is another focus area of Healthy People 2010. The debate over whether or not immunizations can contribute to the ASDs proves to be a barrier to improving health in the United States through immunizations. With or without scientific evidence, parents who choose not to immunize their children will ultimately impact our ability to attain the goals of Healthy People 2010. The scope of this text does not allow for participation in this debate, but to take an objective look at how we can work toward disease prevention and health promotion and what barriers we have to overcome (see http://www.healthypeople.gov/About/hpfact.htm).

CHALLENGES IN NEUROLOGICAL DISORDERS

There are numerous challenges for the patient and practitioner dealing with neurological disorders. Many neurological disorders affect various areas of the physical, emotional, and financial aspect of the patient's life. It would be difficult for the nurse to decide which area needs to be addressed and even more challenging for the patient to make decisions. This particular population may require even more gentle guidance to elicit areas that need improvement. Because depression is often a comorbidity, the patient may have difficulty focusing on the issues at hand. Later we discuss the psychological issues more in depth, but they must be mentioned here because of the significant effect they have on the person with a neurological disorder. Although a challenging task, the use of motivational interviewing techniques can prove to be helpful with each encounter.

Chronic pain puts forth significant hurdles for any patient. It is difficult to understand, and many do not know enough tactics to improve the pain or the pain is resistant to treatment. Pain comes from many sources and is believed to affect 20–30% of the Western population. Management with medication has been found to decrease the level of pain by 30–40% in less than half the patients studied. Typically, patients are first treated for the pain, whether by medication or physical therapy. When pain is not controlled in these areas, patients are forced to look at behaviors they have that may impact the frequency or level of pain. Unfortunately, we have created a society that believes they can go to the doctor and get something to cure their pain. Helping the patient to see that certain behaviors they exhibit can impact the pain can be quite challenging and can evoke resistance. Another challenge related to chronic pain is that it is often a factor in creating additional problems, such as drug/alcohol use and abuse (Turk, Swanson, & Tunks, 2008).

Some neurological disorders leave patients dependent on others because of their disabilities. The focus of the disease management is handled by their caregiver. Individual caregivers may be overwhelmed by providing all the care and challenged to meet all the demands. Some people may have a variety of caregivers, which can make it difficult to maintain consistency in the patient's routine. Finding a way to ensure patients receive the care they need in a consistent manner and allows for patient participation as much as possible can prove to be a difficult mountain to climb.

BENEFITS OF SELF-MANAGEMENT

There are many benefits to promoting self-management skills. Every choice we make is a choice that will impact the management of our health. Knowledge of prevention and healthy behaviors impacts the overall health of our nation. Injury contributes to some neurological disorders, and prevention is the most important aspect of decreasing brain and spinal cord injury. "Injury prevention behavior is shaped not only by individual choices and motivation, knowledge, skills, and attitudes but also by organizational, economic, environmental, and social factors" (Gorin & Arnold, 2006, p. 370). It is important to remember that each patient is influenced by a number of factors in his or her environment that can preclude making unhealthy choices and lead to risky behaviors. "Education and behavioral change strategies are directed mostly toward decreasing the susceptibility of the host to injury by teaching or motivating individuals to behave differently" (Gorin & Arnold, 2006, p. 373). Through motivational interviewing the nurse can help the patient to examine risky health behaviors and potentially make choices to decrease risk for injury.

Remember that motivational interviewing is a style of counseling. William Miller intended this method of communication to be more than a way to address motivational problems. Patients with neurological disorders may be struggling with many changes that must be addressed. Although we would like to give recommendations for what will help the patient, we need to remember that the responsibility to accept those changes and take the appropriate actions to make those changes lies with the patient (Miller & Rollnick, 2002). Many people with neurological disorders have little control over their daily care, and it is important to promote self-management in any area in which they are capable of participating. This gives them an increased sense of self-efficacy, and that improved confidence can help decrease some of the emotional side effects of the neurological disorder.

Chronic pain management requires significant patient participation. Motivational interviewing has been found to be successful in promoting behavior change that can help promote self-management in this particular area. There are many barriers that interfere with pain management. Through therapeutic communication the nurse may be able to elicit some of the reasons a patient may not be able to properly control pain. Reasons can include personal beliefs and fears surrounding pain medication or lack of financial resources to obtain medication and pain management services. By building a rapport with the patient, the nurse can evoke the various behaviors that may be contributing to the patient not being able to reach optimal pain control. When patients have persistent pain, they "become aware of how factors, such as emotional stress, impact their pain; therefore, they might entertain the possibility that they can learn and use self-management techniques to help them adapt to life with a chronic pain condition" (Turk et al., 2008, p. 218).

One study looked at cancer patients and the effects of chronic pain (Fahey et al., 2008). Motivational interviewing was used and practice implications from that study indicated that providers

- Inquire about beliefs and attitudes
- Help the patients recognize discrepancies and problem solve toward resolution
- Encourage patients to explore obstacles preventing them from reaching goals
- Routinely assess patients' level of readiness and suggest stage-appropriate tasks
- Help patients determine priorities and set agendas accordingly
- Establish a concrete task and be sure to follow up
- Take time for communication, especially by listening to what is said
- Ask, do not tell

Pain management is an area where nurses need improvement. Studies have shown that few nurses discuss pain management with pediatric patients. As part of our role, we are obligated to inquire about pain and pain management. This is necessary, even if the patient is a child. Motivational interviewing can be used in this population as well, and the child patient should have a right to participate in this communication. One study found that children require empathy from the nurses. "Working in a partnership with children can positively influence nursing practice as well as research" (Kortesluoma et al., 2008, p. 148). This study reinforces the importance of taking time to establish a rapport, elicit information, and to work in collaboration with the patient.

Often, when patients have mobility problems, it can be challenging for them to go out to doctor visits, support groups, or educational events. Self-management skills are necessary for this population because of the limitations to go out and seek information, and physician visits are too infrequent to be able to manage all aspects of illness. Studies have shown that telephone interventions with nurses can be very effective in educating and motivating patients. One study examined telephone interactions using motivational interviewing with patients who have MS. There were multiple areas that were evaluated such as "physical activity, spiritual growth, stress management, fatigue and mental health" (Bombardier et al., 2008). Patients who participated in motivational interviewing interactions were most likely to report a more significant improvement in these areas. There were five interactions at a total cost of $150-200. Not only was it cost effective, but it also resulted in increased quality of life for the patient (Bombardier et al., 2008).

Dilorio, Reisinger, Yeager, and McCarty (2008) conducted another self-management program via the telephone for patients who had epilepsy. The method of counseling was motivational interviewing. The patients were very sat-isfied with this method of counseling. The study was able to demonstrate the ef-fectiveness of allowing the patient to dictate the path of the conversation. The patient was able to discuss his or her needs to improve self-management with patient satisfaction. When patients enjoy a method of counseling, they are more likely to participate and have a positive outcome (Dilorio et al., 2008).

CASE STUDIES

The following case studies reflect the benefits of using motivational interview-ing techniques with patients with neurological disorders. This is in contrast to interactions without the use of motivational interviewing.

Case Study 1

The patient has been suffering from chronic pain. After exhausting all efforts to manage the pain, he comes to you for help.

Interaction Without Motivational Interviewing

Nurse: Good morning. How have you been feeling?

Patient: Not too good. The pain is getting unbearable and I just don't think I can take it much longer.

Nurse: I see the doctor had prescribed a new pain medication for you at the last visit. That is probably one of the strongest pain medications you could get. I'm surprised it hasn't helped.

Patient: I might not take it like he said.

Nurse: Well, it is important to follow your doctor's instructions or you won't feel better.

Patient: Okay.

Nurse: So, what can I help you with today?

Patient: I can't think of anything else right now.

Nurse: I'm going to recommend you take the medication the doctor gave you and you should be feeling brand new in no time.

Motivational Interviewing Interaction

Nurse: Good morning. How have you been lately?

Patient: Not very good. My pain is out of control.

Nurse: Tell me about what you have been doing to try to control the pain.

Patient: Well, I did physical therapy for awhile, but my insurance benefit for therapy ran out. I try to do the exercises they taught me, but I have so much pain that it is hard to do them. The doctor had given me a new medication at the last visit, but I'm afraid to take it. (Resistance)

Nurse: So, let me understand. You did what physical therapy your insurance plan allowed you to do. It is difficult to follow through with their exercise recommendations because the pain interferes. And the medication your doctor recommended you have not tried because of some fears you have. I'm wondering if you could tell me a little more about your fears.

Patient: My mother was addicted to pain medications and I am scared to death that I'm going to get addicted. I also know that a lot of prescription pain medications can cause you to be foggy and I want to be able to think clearly. It's probably not very rational because I already get foggy and can't focus because the pain is so intense. (Ambivalence)

Nurse: You have obviously put a lot of thought into this and recognize the risks involved in taking pain medication, yet at the same time you see a negative side to staying where you are at with your pain.

Patient: That's right. And the last thing I want to do is repeat what my mother has gone through.

Nurse: You don't want to get addicted.

Patient: No. That is probably my biggest fear besides living with the pain.

Nurse: Fear seems to be your biggest hurdle right now. Could you share with me how you have coped with fears in the past?

Patient: I don't know. I guess I'm the type of person who learns everything I can about something because the more I know, the less I am afraid. Maybe I need to learn more about the medication and my other options. Can you tell me about the medication? (Change talk)

Nurse: I would be happy to.

Discussion

The previous two scenarios provide two different approaches to a similar patient-nurse interaction. The first scenario provides a brief interaction that demonstrates communication not using motivational interviewing. The nurse does not attempt to elicit additional information to further explore the patient's lack of adherence to a recommended medication regime. The nurse chose to dictate the course of action, which leads the patient to become passive and not comfortable voicing concerns. This nurse made assumptions and gave false reassurance. These tactics are not conducive to promoting behavior change.

The second scenario used motivational interviewing skills to examine the patient's perspective of the situation. By remaining nonjudgmental and using open-ended questions and reflections, the nurse was able to elicit information that may not have otherwise been shared. The nurse was interested in learning about the patient's experience. The patient felt comfortable enough to open up about the barriers he had been encountering while dealing with his chronic pain. When the patient was ready, he asked for assistance in better understanding his options, and the nurse was able to share information so he could make informed decisions. There were several directions this conversation could have gone, but the nurse offered gentle guidance to explore the issue of the patient's fears surrounding treatment of the pain. Likely, if the patient had been more focused on the lack of coverage for the physical therapy, the patient would have resisted the guidance and the nurse would have been inclined to help the patient explore other options.

Case Study 2

The patient has Parkinson's disease. There has been a slow decline in her abilities, and she is requiring more assistance as the disease progresses.

Interaction Without Motivational Interviewing

Nurse: Good morning. How are you doing?

Patient: Oh, not so good. I'm having a harder time getting around.

Nurse: When you say a harder time getting around, do you mean with walking, bathing, getting dressed, or other certain tasks?

Patient: I mean I need to ask my husband to help me get bathed and dressed each day.

Nurse: You can talk to your doctor about that. Are you taking all of your medication?

Patient: Yes.

Nurse: Did you go to your therapies?

Patient: Yes.

Nurse: Do you have any other concerns?

Patient: I guess not.

Motivational Interviewing Interaction

Nurse: Good morning. How have you been doing?

Patient: Not very well. I'm having a harder time getting around.

Nurse: Tell me what that means for you.

Patient: I have needed my husband to help me bathe and get dressed each day.

Nurse: That must be difficult for you.

Patient: It is very difficult. I feel so dependent on him.

Nurse: You are used to being the one who takes care of everything.

Patient: Yes. But right now I can't do it. I am ready to give up. (Resistance)

Nurse: You feel helpless.

Patient: Yes, I do. I have never asked for help with anything. I don't know what I can do so I don't need his help.

Nurse: I can see you are struggling with your mobility, but you aren't sure what you can do or what your options may be.

Patient: Yes. I want to do things for myself, but I don't think I could possibly do these things on my own right now. (Ambivalence)

Nurse: Many patients with Parkinson's go through this same struggle as their mobility decreases. Would you like me to share with you some ways that others have told me they have dealt with this?

Patient: I would love to hear some ideas. I am willing to try anything to be more independent. (Change talk)

Discussion

The previous two scenarios represent nontherapeutic communication and therapeutic communication. The first scenario shows a patient who has an obvious concern. The nurse further assessed the complaint and then proceeded with his own agenda. This could have been a perfect opportunity to discuss possible actions that could improve the patient's mobility. The patient began answering quickly and did not feel comfortable offering more information to the nurse. This situation is not unrealistic due to the time constraints in our practice. Too often we miss what the patient is really saying or what the patient's needs may be. We can make more of a difference if we take a few moments to give our undivided attention and work with the patient to improve his or her lifestyle.

The second scenario gives a picture of how motivational interviewing works. The nurse allowed the patient to dictate where the conversation would go. The nurse walked with the patient through resistance, ambivalence, and into change talk. Although not every patient goes through each of these stages, the nurse should be prepared to respond based on where the patient is during that moment (Figure 10-1). The patient felt comfortable talking about her feelings of helplessness, and this was the issue the nurse addressed. With the use of motivational

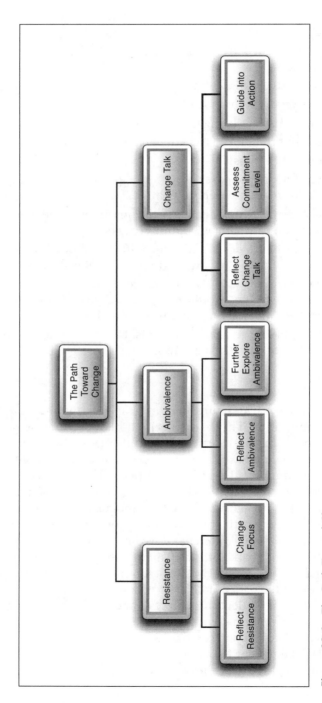

Figure 10-1   The Path Toward Change

interviewing the nurse was able to elicit the patient's need for tools to increase her independence. Once a need was identified, the nurse asked permission to share information that could be helpful rather than telling the patient what to do. This encounter showed the patient and nurse having a conversation, whereas the first scenario was an inquiry.

Case Study 3

The patient has MS, and the medications are not providing a maximum effect. The patient's concern is that the medication changes may make things worse, and she wants to discuss this with the nurse.

Interaction Without Motivational Interviewing

Nurse: Good afternoon. How are you doing today?

Patient: I'm doing okay.

Nurse: Let's take a few moments to go over your medication.

Patient: Okay.

Nurse: I see you are taking Amantadine. Is that correct?

Patient: Yes, I am. I really don't think my medications are working as well as they should. The doctor said I should get relief from some of my symptoms, but they seem to be getting worse.

Nurse: What symptoms are you having?

Patient: The weakness in my hands is getting worse and so is my vision. The doctor said those things should improve now that I'm taking medication.

Nurse: The dose is the typical starting dose and you just need to give it some time.

Patient: Okay.

Motivational Interviewing Interaction

Nurse: Good afternoon. How are you doing today?

Patient: I'm doing okay.

Nurse: What can we do to make you better than okay?

Patient: I don't know. The doctor gave me some medications and my symptoms are getting worse instead of better.

Nurse: You were hoping to see improvement by now.

Patient: Yes. I don't understand why the medications aren't working. I know the doctor said there is another medication to add if needed, but I don't know.

Nurse: It can be difficult getting the symptoms under control and finding the right medication doses and combinations. This must be frustrating for you.

Patient: It is very frustrating. I want a quick fix and don't want to take so many medications that I have problems with side effects on top of everything else. (Ambivalence)

Nurse: You feel like you are in limbo waiting for the medication to work and are hesitant to add anything because of possible side effects. How can I help you?

Patient: Just listening helps. Maybe helping me to better understand the medications and what to expect so I'm not so anxious to see improvements.

Nurse: I would be happy to talk with you about the medications and possibly some things you could do while you are getting stabilized with the medications.

Patient: That would be great. If there is anything I can do for myself I want to know so I can help things along. (Change talk)

Discussion

In these two scenarios the patient presents to the nurse with concerns that her medications are not working as she thought they should. The nurse disregards the patient's concern and pacifies her by saying it will take some time. This patient may have not been taking her medication correctly, may not understand the effects of the medication, or could even be suffering from anxiety as a result of a new diagnosis of MS. The nurse did not take the time to further assess or elicit information to better understand the patient's concern. The nurse would have been more effective in helping the patient if she had listened and helped resolve any ambivalence the patient was experiencing.

The second scenario demonstrates how an interaction can go by using motivational interviewing techniques. The nurse inquired about what the patient needed. The patient was clear about her concerns, and the nurse was able to easily address them. The nurse did not have a preset agenda and allowed the patient to determine the path of the conversation. The nurse simply asked the patient how she could help her and this left the door open for the patient to voice her concerns. There was not any resistance from the patient because the nurse was not forcing anything on her. The patient was ambivalent about the medications, and with the nurse's guidance she was able to resolve that ambivalence.

PRACTICE TOOLS (FIGURE 10-2)

1. It is important to recognize when the patient becomes passive. This should give the nurse an indication that she could change the approach to be more effective. When the nurse is taking control of the conversation and telling the patient what to do, the patient will often respond passively, with short answers. When the nurse is not listening to what the patient is saying, the patient will become passive. The goal is to bring information out of the patient to help him or her make the necessary self-discoveries, explore options, and decide what actions, if any, should be taken (Rollnick, Miller, & Butler, 2008).

2. Some patients with neurological disorders depend on others for their daily care. It is important to allow the patient to participate in decision making as much as possible. Just as important is the participation of the

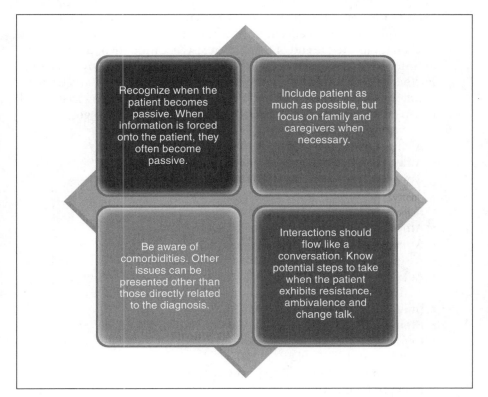

Figure 9-2 Practice Tools

caregiver because he or she has challenges in providing care. To improve a patient's quality of life, decrease risk factors, or, in the very least, maintain current health status, the nurse must include all those involved.

3. Many neurological disorders come with comorbidities. During any encounter the patient may be more concerned about issues other than the direct care of the neurological disorder. Knowing about other issues that can exist for this population is very important. This knowledge will prepare you for some topics that may be the focus of the conversation.

4. Some interactions go smoothly like a conversation. Other times, the nurse must make decisions about how best to respond. There are no perfect answers and there is more than one way to approach every situation. As noted in Figure 10-1, when the patient exhibits resistance the nurse can either reflect resistance or attempt to change the focus through reflections, metaphors, additional open-ended questions, or simple silence. When the patient is ambivalent, the nurse can reflect that ambivalence back to the patient or further explore that ambivalence through open-ended questions and reflections. It is not safe to assume that statements of change talk are the end of the challenge. Once the patient demonstrates an interest in change, it does not mean the patient is ready to change. Further exploration about commitment to change is necessary. Each encounter is a new adventure, with the path dimly lit, requiring us to use all of our senses to find our way to where the patient wants to go.

5. Use available resources:
   - Alzheimer's Association
   - American Academy of Neurology
   - American Autoimmune Related Diseases Association
   - American Parkinson Disease Association
   - American Pediatric Association
   - American Neurological Association
   - Amyotrophic Lateral Sclerosis Association
   - Association for Behavioral Analysis International
   - Autism Society of America
   - Autism Speaks
   - Brain Injury Association of America
   - Brain Trauma Foundation
   - Centers for Disease Control and Prevention
   - Child Neurology Society
   - Christopher and Dana Reeve Foundation
   - Epilepsy Foundation
   - Multiple Sclerosis Association of America
   - Multiple Sclerosis Foundation

- Muscular Dystrophy Association
- National Center for Injury Prevention & Control
- National Center on Birth Defects and Developmental Disabilities
- National Institute of Child Health and Human Development
- National Institute of Neurological Disorders
- National Multiple Sclerosis Society
- National Parkinson Foundation
- National Spinal Cord Injury Association
- Spinal Cord Society
- The Michael J. Fox Foundation for Parkinson's Research

TAKE-AWAY POINTS

1. Neurological disorders can be devastating, not only to the patients afflicted but also to the families, caregivers, and community at large. Quality of life can be significantly diminished, and our role as nurses requires us to help the patient improve quality of life through health promotion, disease prevention, and health maintenance. Motivational interviewing is an essential tool that can help us accomplish this.
2. Studies have proven motivational interviewing to be effective in areas of chronic illness, MS, chronic pain management, and epilepsy. Results from many of these studies can be transferred to other neurological disorders. Although more research is needed, studies have shown promise that motivational interviewing holds for our future in promoting behavior change.
3. "Nonadherence" and "noncompliance" radiates a negative connotation. What we need to be aware of is that patients who have been given these titles have many reasons for not following through with recommendations, such as taking medication as ordered. Sometimes, they simply lack knowledge. When that is established, asking permission to share information shows respect, and the patient is often open to listening. There are a number of other reasons not to follow recommendations, such as financial constraints, religious beliefs, other disabilities can interfere, fears, and denial. Allow the patient to explore the barriers and take an objective look at the patient's reasoning. Remain nonjudgmental. With the proper guidance, they can determine if they need to change their perspective and/or actions.
4. In following Healthy People 2010 goals, we must work toward prevention of injuries and providing accurate information regarding immunizations. Every patient encounter gives us the opportunity to work toward these goals. Being aware of the impact that injuries, such as brain injuries and spinal cord injuries, can have on the health of our country will help us to incorporate prevention into our encounters when appropriate.

SUMMARY

This chapter addresses issues in neurological health and ways that motivational interviewing can improve each encounter. We strive to help this particular population to maintain health, decrease risk factors, and improve quality of life. As more research is performed, the results will likely support what has already been proven, that motivational interviewing is an effective tool used to promote behavior change, to help patients to have an active role in decision making, and to help us to take steps toward a healthier nation.

REFERENCES

Alzheimer's Association. (2009). 2009 Alzheimer's disease facts and figures: Executive summary.

Bombardier, C., Cunniffe, M., Wadhwani, R., Gibbons, L., Blake, K., & Kraft, G. (2008). The efficacy of telephone counseling for health promotion in people with multiple sclerosis: A randomized controlled trial. *Archives of Physical Medicine and Rehabilitation, 89,* 1849–1856.

Dilorio, C., Reisinger, E., Yeager, K., & McCarty, F. (2008). A telephone-based self-management program for people with epilepsy. *Epilepsy & Behavior, 14,* 232–236.

Fahey, K., Rao, S., Douglas, M., Thomas, M., Elliott, J., & Miaskowski, C. (2008). Nurse coaching to explore and modify patient attitudinal barriers interfering with effective cancer pain management. *Oncology Nursing Forum, 35*(2), 233–240.

Farley, T. (2004). Amyotrophic lateral sclerosis. Arkansas Spinal Cord Commission. August.

Gorin, S., & Arnold, J. (2006). *Health promotion in practice.* San Francisco: Jossey-Bass.

Kortesluoma, R., Nikkonen, M., & Serlo, W. (2008). "You just have to make the pain go away"- Children's experiences of pain management. *Pain Management Nursing, 9*(4), 143–149.

Miller, W., & Rollnick, S. (2002). *Motivational interviewing: Preparing people for change* (2nd ed.). New York: The Guilford Press.

Rollnick, S., Miller, W., & Butler, C. (2008). *Motivational interviewing in health care: Helping patients change behavior.* New York: The Guilford Press.

Turk, D., Swanson, K., & Tunks, E. (2008). Psychological approaches in the treatment of chronic pain patients—When pills, scalpels, and needles are not enough.

CHAPTER 11

Motivational Interviewing in Musculoskeletal Disorders

INTRODUCTION

Musculoskeletal disorders include disorders of the bones, joints, and connective tissue. This group of disorders is varied and can be complicated by issues such as chronic pain. Many people are afflicted at some point in their life by a musculoskeletal disorder, if even by a simple sprain or strain. "Bone and joint disorders impair daily activities more than other medical conditions" (see http://www.onepatient.us/theFacts/needForCare02.cfm). Decreased mobility or immobility can lead to a number of other issues such as pneumonia, skin ulcers, increased pain, decreased range of motion, and increased risk for weight gain.

The ability to move without discomfort is often taken for granted until we suffer from a disorder of the musculoskeletal system.

In 2005 the National Center for Health Statistics published the following data (see http://www.onepatient.us/theFacts/needForCare02.cfm):

- 62 million American adults suffer from low back pain.
- 32.3 million American adults suffer from neck pain.
- 58.9 million American adults suffer from chronic joint pain.
- 46.9 million American adults were diagnosed with arthritis.
- Prescription medications for bone and joint pain increased by 50% from 1998 to 2004.
- There were 437 million work days lost due to bone pain and arthritis.

Clearly, musculoskeletal health is important to maintain due to the number of people affected. The cost of missed work is a good indicator that we need to be promoting musculoskeletal health. Other costs to consider are medication, physician visits, and physical and occupational therapies. Information about musculoskeletal disorders and connective tissue disorders is limited compared with information researched for other chapters in this text, but musculoskeletal disorders have a significant impact on quality of life for the individual. Without proper education, self-management tools, and support patients will certainly suffer needlessly. We continue by giving statistics for a variety of musculoskeletal and connective tissue disorders.

Osteoporosis is a disease that leads to fragile bones and increased risk of fractures. Approximately 10 million Americans have osteoporosis, yet 34 million have, "low bone mass," a precursor to osteoporosis. Women are more at risk than men. This disease can occur at any age and is responsible for more than 1.5 million fractures yearly. It is estimated that $14 billion are spent each year for osteoporosis and related fractures (see http://www.niams.nih.gov/Health_Info/Bone/Osteoporosis/default.asp).

Arthritis is a group of disorders that contributes to pain, stiffness, and swelling in and around the joints. The most common form of arthritis is **osteoarthritis**, but **rheumatoid arthritis (RA)**, fibromyalgia, and lupus are also included in this category. Lupus and RA not only affect the joints but can also affect multiple other organ systems. Approximately one in five American adults has some form of arthritis. By 2030 it is predicted that 67 million adults will be afflicted, with more than one-third suffering limited mobility as a result. One in every 250 children is also affected. Arthritis is a common cause of disability and is linked to many work-related limitations. Work-related losses in 2003 were approximately $47 billion. Direct costs of arthritis in 2003 were about $81 billion. Arthritis is a debilitating constellation of disorders that has a significant impact on the health of our nation (see http://www.cdc.gov/nccdphp/publications/aag/arthritis.htm).

Rheumatoid arthritis is an inflammatory disease of the joints, which can severely limit mobility. There are an estimated 1.3 million people with RA. Although the overall rate is decreasing, the number of older people being diagnosed is increasing. Two to three times more women than men are diagnosed. As previously noted, this disorder may not only involve the joints but can contribute to fatigue; problems with red blood cells, such as anemia or decrease in production of the cells; dry eyes and mouth; or neck pain. There are other more rare symptoms, and potential side effects of medication used to treat RA that can only complicate matters more (see http://www.niams.nih.gov/Health_Info/Rheumatic_Disease/default.asp).

Osteoarthritis is a condition that causes a breakdown of the cartilage between the joints. Twenty-seven million Americans are affected. Most often, the symptoms present after age 40 with slow progression. Individual costs associated with RA are estimated at $5,700 per person per year. Considering the number of people in our population affected, this is a costly disease. Although some risk factors are not modifiable, weight loss and routine exercise can decrease the risk of osteoarthritis (Arthritis Foundation, 2008).

Paget's disease is a disorder that causes bones to grow larger and weaker than average. The bones become misshapen and fracture more easily. Typically, this occurs in only one bone of the body, most likely the pelvis, spine, legs, or skull. Approximately 1 million people in the United States suffer from this disease. It is most common in older people, aged 45–74. Men are more likely than women to have this disease. Many people who have Paget's disease also have some form of arthritis. There is no known way to prevent this disease, so the focus is on management (see http://www.niams.nih.gov/Health_Info/Bone/ Pagets/default.asp).

Osteogenesis imperfecta is a genetic disorder that causes the bones to be brittle. Eight forms of osteogenesis imperfecta have been identified. These forms vary in when fractures typically occur and can range from mild to severe. A mild form may not have many fractures occur. The most severe is lethal. In some cases fractures occur in the womb. Some children do not survive because of severe bone deformities and impact on the respiratory system. There are no statistics to tell how many people are afflicted, but an estimated 20,000 to 50,000 Americans are believed to be afflicted (see http://www.niams.nih.gov/Health_Info/Bone/Osteogenesis_Imperfecta/default.asp).

Polymyalgia rheumatica is a rheumatic disorder that is related to musculoskeletal pain and stiffness. Areas affected are typically the neck, shoulder, and hip regions. The population affected is over the age of 50. The symptoms usually resolve within 1–2 years. Symptoms can be controlled with corticosteroids. Often, polymyalgia rheumatica and giant cell arteritis occur at the same time. This results in inflammation of the temporal, other scalp, neck, and arm arteries. The arteries narrow and block blood flow, which could lead to more serious problems, such as vision loss or stroke. Giant cell arteritis affects approximately

200 out of every 100,000 people over the age of 50 (see http://www.niams.nih. gov/Health_Info/Polymyalgia/default.asp).

Fibromyalgia is another chronic disorder that causes pain and tenderness of the musculoskeletal system and connective tissues. It does not involve the joints or cause inflammation. Unfortunately, it also causes fatigue, sleep problems, morning stiffness, painful menstruation, memory problems ("fibro fog"), headaches, irritable bowel syndrome, and sensitivities to light and sound. There is an estimated 5 million people over the age of 18 diagnosed in the United States. Approximately 80–90% of those with fibromyalgia are women. Most people are diagnosed during middle adulthood but often have symptoms earlier in life. Even children can be affected. It has been noted that people with some rheumatic diseases are at higher risk for fibromyalgia. This disorder is often difficult to treat and can have patients suffering with pain and fatigue until the right treatment regimen is found. They then are dealing with chronic pain issues, as discussed in Chapter 10 (see http://www.niams.nih.gov/Health_ Info/Fibromyalgia/default.asp).

Musculoskeletal disorders often present with pain as the primary symptom and lead to some form of physical disability. Patients who suffer from musculoskeletal disorders are often misunderstood and not properly treated by the healthcare provider. It is estimated that 60% of people on long-term sick leave or who have retired early did so because of chronic musculoskeletal conditions. During the last 5 years, $254 billion have been spent in the United States on costs related to musculoskeletal disorders. The financial impact, along with individual consequences, work-related disabilities, and the future of our nation's health, has led us to focus on the pain that accompanies musculoskeletal disorders. The Joint Commission on Accreditation of Healthcare Organizations has identified pain as the fifth vital sign. This places an emphasis on increased understanding, thorough assessment of, and proper treatment of musculoskeletal pain. "The monumental impact of musculoskeletal conditions is now recognized by the United Nations, the World Health Organization, World Bank, and numerous governments throughout the world through support of the Bone and Joint Decade 2000 to 2010 initiative" (Walsh et al., 2008, p. 1830). This initiative provides standards of care for acute and chronic pain with musculoskeletal issues and places an emphasis on pain management (Figure 11-1). Improved prevention, assessment, management, and evaluation is needed, and this initiative offers ways to accomplish these tasks.

Musculoskeletal injuries are very common. It is estimated that more than 25,000 Americans sprain their ankle each day, and this is one of the most common injuries. The **National Institute for Occupational Safety and Health** reports that most musculoskeletal injuries occur as a result of overexertion and repetitive motions. Injuries can occur due to sports, work, and accidents. A de-

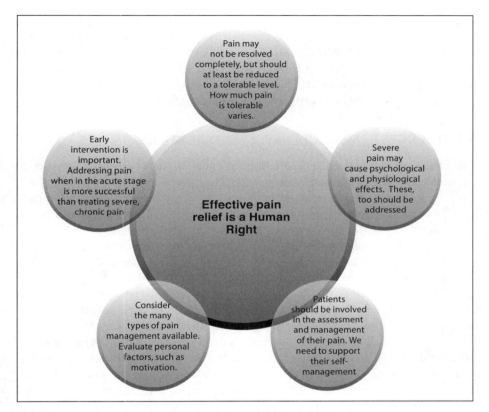

Figure 11-1   The Bone and Joint Decade 2000–2010 Initiative

Source: Adapted from Walsh, N., et al., 2008.

tailed breakdown of these statistics is not available. A need for updated data can help put this into perspective. The important point is injuries can be prevented (see http://cdc.gov/niosh/docs/97-141/ and http://www.niams.nih.gov/Health_Info/Sprains_Strains/default.asp).

In our goal to achieve a healthier nation, Healthy People 2010 has designated a focus area for arthritis, osteoporosis, chronic back conditions, and occupational safety and health. There is also a focus area for injury and violence prevention, which can include musculoskeletal injuries. Injuries can be prevented by a variety of measures, such as protective equipment, safe work and play areas, and proper use of equipment. There were approximately 2.1 million injuries and illness in the workplace in 2006. Many, if not all, could have been prevented. Our role as healthcare providers is significant in promoting prevention to decrease the incidence of musculoskeletal injuries. Disability and secondary conditions is another focus area for Healthy People 2010. Musculoskeletal disorders are another common cause for disability, and some of the secondary conditions may be skin ulcers, obesity, pneumonia, increased pain, and decreased mobility caused by the musculoskeletal disorder (National Center for Health Statistics, 2009; see http://www.healthypeople.gov/About/hpfact.htm).

CHALLENGES IN MUSCULOSKELETAL DISORDERS

Management of any disease or disorder has challenges. The primary challenge in managing musculoskeletal disorders is that they are often misunderstood. Pain, being the most common symptom to bring a patient to the doctor, cannot be seen. It is felt by the patient, and their personal pain threshold is not comparable with others. With stories of "drug-seeking" patients who complain of pain to get high off the medications, it leaves the practitioner in a difficult position. How do we know when patients are being honest about their pain? How do we know their pain is at a level that may require a controlled substance? We must build a rapport with our patients so they can build trust in us and we can build trust in them. Once that is established, a more effective working relationship is formed and pain management will commence.

Pain is often difficult for the patient to describe. Pinpointing a location and determining if it is joint, muscular, bone, tendon, or ligament pain can be difficult. A thorough examination is necessary. Description of the pain, such as location, time of onset, constant versus intermittent, stabbing versus dull, and relieving and aggravating factors should be assessed. Early treatment of acute pain prevents complications of treatment often seen when a patient has severe pain. It can be very difficult to control or even decrease if the patient does not have symptoms managed early after diagnosis of the musculoskeletal problem.

Other challenges include complications from the decreased mobility that is often experienced when there is a musculoskeletal disorder. Outcomes can include skin ulcers caused from pressure when lying in bed and decreased exercise due to immobility that can lead to obesity, muscle wasting, decreased digestion, increased fatigue from lack of exercise, and increased pain with stiffness of joints. Any one of these issues may be a priority for the patient, and the use of motivational interviewing can help overcome some of these challenges.

BENEFITS OF SELF-MANAGEMENT

Self-management skills are important for anyone afflicted by one of the many musculoskeletal disorders. Patient participation in pain management, scheduling of exercise, or therapies can give the patient some independence and increase self-confidence. With increased self-confidence, there is often increased participation in care. Learning self-management is not only important for the individual but will also help to meet the goals set before us by Healthy People 2010. Specifically, there are three objectives related to arthritis self-management:

1. Arthritis education
2. Weight counseling
3. Physical activity counseling

The Arthritis Foundation and the Centers for Disease Control and Prevention combined efforts to provide a program that addresses exercise, aquatics, and self-help courses. There was progress in the categories of weight and physical activity counseling in 2002 and 2003, but arthritis education was not as successful. "Education is the 'portal' through which a person with arthritis must go to achieve successful self-management" (Koehn & Esdaile, 2008, p. 397).

When diagnosed with arthritis, or any chronic disease, patients are not likely to have a complete understanding of what can be done for their condition and what tools may be used to improve their condition. Keep in mind that the patient may have provided care for a family member with the same condition or have a strong background of knowledge in the area. When we use motivational interviewing, we can assess their current knowledge and offer guidance in areas where they have less knowledge. Supporting a person in self-management includes providing information. Within the guiding style of motivational interviewing, information should be provided with permission from the patient (Rollnick, Miller, & Butler, 2008).

One study looked at self-management in patients with arthritis and found that patients had different levels of involvement in their self-management. The reason for this was that patients are all at different stages of change. The transtheoretical model of change was used in this study. Patients were evaluated and placed into groups of precontemplation, contemplation, preparation, unprepared action, and prepared maintenance. The findings of this study supported the need to evaluate how ready a patient is to change in order to be successful in promoting self-management skills (Keefe et al., 2000). By using motivational interviewing tactics within our practice, we do just that. "The first step is to ask about the importance of change and then, if it seems appropriate, to elicit a numerical rating" (Rollnick et al., 2008, p. 60). This is the readiness ruler that incorporates the Likert scale from 1 to 10. This scale can provide a wealth of information. When a patient gives a number, you may have a basic idea of where they are but not really why they are there. Asking patients why they aren't at a lower number on the scale can open up clues to their confidence level, barriers they perceive, or accomplishments they have already made. Another approach is to ask them what it will take to get them further up the scale. This encourages the patient to take a thoughtful look at where they are, where they want to be, and what is standing in the way of getting there.

Health promotion is a significant factor in our role as nurses. Promotion of healthy lifestyles can improve the health of those with musculoskeletal disorders. Some recommendations for health promotion are as follows (Bergman 2007):

- Physical activity and improved muscle strength
- Avoid smoking
- Maintaining normal body weight
- Dietary recommendations for calcium and vitamin D
- Safe work environments and activities

Each area can be included in self-management education.

Medication adherence is often a problem yet is a large part of self-management. Elliott (2008) looked at adherence to medications in the treatment of RA. The author noted that adherence to medications in this population is often less than 50%. The reasons are many, but obviously this is a problem because the symptoms are uncontrolled. The medications will not cure RA but can help with symptoms and delay the progression of the disease. This review reported that "educational interventions have had limited effectiveness in changing behavior because of the limited ability of changes in knowledge to produce lasting behavioral change" (Elliott, 2008, p. 14). Simply providing knowledge will not promote behavior change. Motivational interviewing allows the provider to investigate the barriers and support the patient as he or she explores options, weighs the pros and cons, and determines the best option at that time. Patients are more likely to change behaviors when they determine their actions are hurting themselves. By providing information about the medications, we are telling them what they need, when in fact they need to decide for themselves, based on their current financial, health, and psychosocial situation.

Two separate articles focused on fibromyalgia and the various disorders that tend to be a part of the fibromyalgia syndrome (Sarzi-Puttini, Buskila, Carrabba, Doria, & Atzeni, 2008; Yunus, 2007). This is an interesting disorder in that there are no standardized treatments because the musculoskeletal pain is often accompanied by other health issues, such as irritable bowel syndrome, chronic fatigue, headaches, and mood disorders. Both articles stress the importance of treating these particular patients as individuals with different biological and psychosocial issues that impact the overall presentation of the patient. The complexity of this disorder prompts individualization, when in fact this individualization should be considered in every encounter with every patient, regardless of the diagnosis. Self-management tools that are recommended include the use of exercise, physical therapy, stress management, biofeedback, and medications. With motivational interviewing these options can be explored, allowing the patient to determine what he or she is willing and/or able to try (Sarzi-Puttini et al., 2008; Yunus, 2007).

CASE STUDIES

The following case studies demonstrate the difference between a non-motivational interviewing interaction and a motivational interviewing interaction with patients suffering from various musculoskeletal disorders.

Case Study 1

The patient has a recurrent knee injury. The patient has not given up any of the activities that contribute to this repetitive injury.

Interaction Without Motivational Interviewing

Nurse: Good morning. How are you doing today?

Patient: Well, honestly, I'm tired of coming in here about this knee.

Nurse: So, you have injured it again?

Patient: Yes.

Nurse: How did it happen this time?

Patient: Well, I was playing football with some friends and I got tackled and it twisted.

Nurse: I see your last injury was only 2 weeks ago. You really need to give your knee a rest so it has time to heal.

Patient: It was feeling better, so I didn't think it was a problem.

Nurse: Well, you should follow the doctor's recommendation to rest the knee for the next 4 weeks and then let her recheck it before you start up the activity again. You must know that you may be causing permanent damage to your knee.

Patient: No, I didn't know that. I guess I'll try to rest it.

Motivational Interviewing Interaction

Nurse: Good morning. How are you doing today?

Patient: Not good. I'm tired of injuring my knee.

Nurse: I see you were here about 2 weeks ago with an injury of that same knee. Could you tell me what happened?

Patient: Well, I did what the doctor told me and it was feeling better. So, I was playing football with some friends yesterday and got tackled. When I went down, it twisted and now I'm having a hard time walking on it.

Nurse: Many people feel they must be healed if they are feeling better, but that is not always the case. A re-injury is common if activity is started too soon. What are your thoughts about that?

Patient: Well, I did feel better, so why wouldn't I think it was healed? (Resistance)

Nurse: In many situations, feeling better tells us our body has healed, but when we injure a joint, it is not always that easy. It can be difficult because you can't see the healing process inside the joint.

Patient: So, you are saying that my knee wasn't even healed?

Nurse: That is very likely and may be why you received another injury so quickly.

Patient: My mother said I need to stop playing football, but I'm not going to do that.

Nurse: (silent.)

Patient: I love football and it's the one thing I really enjoy. (Ambivalence)

Nurse: On one hand, you love football and want to continue playing, but on the other hand, you keep getting injured, which could ultimately prevent you from playing football or other sports in the future.

Patient: I didn't think of it like that. What can I do to prevent another injury? (Change talk)

Nurse: We can go over a few things that may help if you would like.

Patient: Yes, I would. I don't want to take a chance that I won't ever play again.

Nurse: On a scale of 1 to 10, how committed are you to preventing another injury?

Patient: I would say about a 9 or 10.

Nurse: You are very motivated.

Patient: Yes, I am determined not to have another injury.

Discussion

In the previous two scenarios the patient was not following recommendations for treatment, and this resulted in repetitive injury of his knee. In the first scenario the nurse was accusatory and the patient was on the defensive about how it happened and that he really did not know he needed to continue to rest the knee once it felt better. Often, there are misunderstandings when patients receive instructions for self-management. It is extremely important to evaluate a patient's level of understanding after any information is provided.

In the second scenario the nurse allows the patient to direct the conversation. The patient is ambivalent about giving up football yet does not want to repeat his injury. The nurse used the Likert scale to determine how motivated the patient was to work toward injury prevention. When the patient reported he was at the top of the scale, the nurse saw little room for improvement or movement forward. This patient was clearly ready to make behavior changes to decrease his risk for injury.

Case Study 2

The patient has RA and has been suffering from a flare-up of symptoms. The patient is looking for pain relief.

Interaction Without Motivational Interviewing

Nurse: Good morning. How have you been since our last visit?

Patient: I was doing fine, and then over the past week my joints are so swollen and painful.

Nurse: Okay. Have there been any changes in your routine or medications?

Patient: Well, because of the pain, I'm not as active now. I also find the medications make me feel terrible.

Nurse: So, you aren't taking your medication?

Patient: No, I just can't tolerate them. I need something that doesn't make me feel so sick.

Nurse: Unfortunately, a lot of the medications to treat rheumatoid arthritis have a lot of side effects that are uncomfortable. But, I'll let you talk to the doctor about it.

Patient: Okay.

Nurse: Now, about the activity, if you can keep active, that will help a lot.

Patient: Right.

Nurse: I would recommend at least ½ hour of activity daily. Something like swimming or riding a bike.

Patient: I might consider it if I weren't in so much pain.

Nurse: It is important to understand that activity can actually help with the pain management.

Patient: Okay.

Motivational Interviewing Interaction

Nurse: Good morning. How have you been doing?

Patient: Not so good. I have been having more pain and swelling in my joints again.

Nurse: What, if anything, can you say has been different in your routine?

Patient: Well, I like to exercise, but I have been in so much pain that I just can't exercise every day like I was. And the medications are making me feel terrible.

Nurse: So, the exercise has been limited, and you are having a difficult time with side effects of the medication.

Patient: That's right. I would have horrible abdominal cramps and headaches. So, I stopped taking them. Now those symptoms are better, but I'm back to the joint pain and swelling. I just can't win! (Ambivalence)

Nurse: You are very frustrated.

Patient: Yes, I am. I wish I could feel better. (Change talk)

Nurse: Trying different medication that the doctor may recommend may be helpful. In addition, there may be some things you can do at home to help manage.

Patient: I'd like to hear about what I can do.

Nurse: Physical therapy can offer some helpful ways to manage the pain and mobility. They often help you to exercise and use water therapy. This is something you can also do at home if you have a pool.

Patient: I do have a pool. Maybe I could try that.

Nurse: On a scale of 1 to 10, how motivated are you to make some changes to help your mobility?

Patient: Honestly, I would have to say about a 6 or 7.

Nurse: So, there is some motivation. What makes you a 6 or 7, rather than a 3 or 4?

Patient: Well, I want to try the things you offer, but at the same time I'm not sure how well I can do it because of the pain I'm in.

Nurse: What would it take to get you to an 8 or a 9?

Patient: Pain relief! If the doctor could give me something to help with the pain, I will be able to exercise more routinely.

Discussion

In the previous two scenarios the patient and nurse were addressing issues of pain management in RA. Nonadherence to medication is common in this group as previously discussed. In the first scenario, the nurse did not further explore the patient's concerns and disregarded the fact that pain was limiting her mobility. Instead, the nurse tried to push the patient to exercise despite the pain. The patient became passive and was not likely to go home and exercise. Instead, this patient is likely to go home and continue to suffer with her pain.

In the second scenario the nurse elicits more information from the patient to better understand the barriers she is facing. They discussed the medications, and the nurse explained that there are other options for medications. The nurse also offered other methods to help, and the patient thought the use of her pool may be worth trying to increase her mobility. The nurse used the Likert scale to get a better understanding of how motivated this patient is to move forward and try some things to help herself and found that pain management will help the patient to achieve her goals. There are many situations when use of the Likert scale is beneficial and this scenario demonstrated effective use.

Case Study 3

The patient has fibromyalgia and is suffering from musculoskeletal pain as well as chronic fatigue and depression.

Interaction Without Motivational Interviewing

Nurse: Good morning. How are you today?

Patient: Okay, I guess.

Nurse: I see you are here following up for your fibromyalgia. How has that been?

Patient: I hurt all over.

Nurse: I'm sorry to hear that. Tell me what you have been doing to manage the discomfort.

Patient: Nothing. Nothing seems to help. I've given up.

Nurse: There is no need to give up. There are plenty of things to do that can help you feel better.

Patient: Like what?

Nurse: Medications . . .

Patient: They aren't working.

Nurse: Physical therapy . . .

Patient: Tried that and my insurance benefit ran out.

Nurse: Massage . . .

Patient: I can't afford it, nor do I have time to go get a massage!

Nurse: Exercise . . .

Patient: Are you crazy? I can barely move, much less exercise.

Nurse: I can see you have tried a lot of things. Maybe the doctor has some other ideas for you.

Motivational Interviewing Interaction

Nurse: Good morning. How are you doing?

Patient: Okay, I guess.

Nurse: What is getting in the way of your being good, or even great?

Patient: I just feel horrible all the time. I hurt all over.

Nurse: The pain is almost unbearable.

Patient: It is unbearable. I just can't take it!

Nurse: You feel helpless.

Patient: That's exactly how I feel.

Nurse: Many people with fibromyalgia feel that way. Tell me a little about how it's affecting you.

Patient: Well, I am so exhausted, but I can't sleep. It hurts to move and it hurts to lay down for any length of time. I just want to lay there and cry.

Nurse: I remember that you also have chronic fatigue, which is common with fibromyalgia. Being exhausted and having chronic pain can cause some people to feel depressed. What are your thoughts about that?

Patient: If you are asking if I feel depressed, I guess I would have to say yes. I want to cry all the time and everything just feels hopeless. I feel like I have no control over anything anymore.

Nurse: Tell me a little more about that.

Patient: I cry at least three times a day. Sometimes there is no reason that I can tell. Maybe it's the pain, but sometimes I will just burst out crying. My husband thinks I'm crazy.

Nurse: The word "crazy"–what does that mean to you?

Patient: It means my emotions are out of control. I am out of control.

Nurse: You feel you have no control over your situation right now.

Patient: I don't really. And I don't know how much more I can live like this.

Nurse: You don't have to live like this. If there was one thing you could change, what would that be?

Patient: I would not feel so out of control.

Nurse: I'm curious what your thoughts are about how you might improve this situation.

Patient: I don't know really. I read about one of the medications that can be used to treat the fibromyalgia pain that is also for depression. I was hoping to talk to the doctor about that.

Nurse: Yes, Cymbalta has been found to be effective in managing symptoms of both problems. That might be the best place to start.

Patient: That is the only option I know of right now.

Nurse: I have learned a lot from other patients in your situation and ways they found to help with their combination of symptoms. Would you like me to share some of those options with you?

Patient: I would love for you to. I need all the help I can get right now.

Discussion

In the previous two scenarios the patient has a variety of issues surrounding the fibromyalgia and other disorders that often coexist with fibromyalgia. In the first scenario the patient has exhausted the tools she had available to manage the musculoskeletal pain at home. The patient is resistant to each option the nurse offers until the nurse gives up and passes the issue onto the physician. This would typically be a situation the nurse could discuss with the patient, but the nurse was faced with resistance and chose to back down from the resistance.

In the second scenario the nurse not only talked with the patient about the fibromyalgia, but also elicited enough information to determine that this patient is also depressed, a common comorbidity. With this discovery the nurse was able to help the patient see the importance of addressing the depression as well as the pain. The nurse remained nonjudgmental, which allowed the patient to open up about the depression symptoms and explore how the combination of symptoms is impacting her life. The patient had already decided one treatment that could help her situation and intended to discuss this with the physician. The nurse offered validation of feelings the patient was experiencing and, with permission, offered additional methods to help with symptoms. The use of motivational interviewing was beneficial in this interaction because it brought out patient issues that may otherwise have gone untreated, decreasing the patient's quality of life.

PRACTICE TOOLS (FIGURE 11-2)

1. It is important to recognize that patients with musculoskeletal disorders often suffer from pain. With this pain comes controversy over the existence of that pain, the best methods of treatment, and patient involvement in care. All patients have a "right" to pain management. When pain is not properly managed, the patient continues to return over and over again,

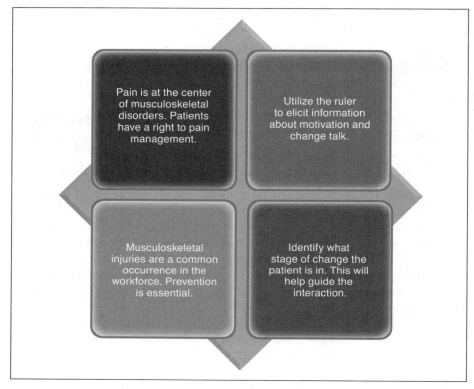

Figure 11-2   Practice Tools

seeking assistance. As noted in the Bone and Joint Decade 2000–2010 (Walsh et al., 2008), patients have a role in self-management of that pain as well as a need to have assistance from healthcare providers to provide what pain management can get the patient to a tolerable level of pain, if not resolution of pain.

2. Use of a Likert scale or ruler is not new to nursing practice. We use this most often when assessing a patient's level of pain. "Within MI, rulers have a dual purpose. They not only tell you about the patient's motivation but can also elicit change talk" (Rollnick et al., 2008 p. 58). This was demonstrated in the case studies in this chapter. When properly used the ruler can provide information that might otherwise not been offered by the patient. This information can be useful to the nurse because of the depth of information it provides. It is also useful for the patient to further explore his or her issues and help the patient to gain perspective.

3. Patients with musculoskeletal disorders often suffer from decreased mobility. This loss of independence can be devastating to the patient and family. The impact on the workforce is also astounding. In 2001 musculoskeletal injuries accounted for an average 8 workdays missed, compared with 6 workdays for nonfatal injuries and illness. With prevention a priority, there was a decline in cases from 784,145 in 1992 to 522,528 in 2001. This is an example of how prevention can improve the health of our nation (http://www.cdc.gov/niosh/nas/mining/pdfs/2004-146.pdf).

4. Recognizing where the patient is on the continuum of the stages of change provides insight to where the patient has been and where they need to go. For example, if the patient has not even considered his or her options, this patient is in precontemplation and needs to explore options. The patient may be already contemplating making some changes but has not yet decided a path to take. "The most obvious connection between motivational interviewing and the stages of change is that motivational interviewing is an excellent counseling style to use with clients who are in the early stages" (Miller & Rollnick, 2002, p. 202).

5. Use available resources:
   - American Academy of Orthopaedic Surgeons
   - American College of Rheumatology
   - American Orthopedic Society for Sports Medicine
   - American Osteopathic Association
   - American Physical Therapy Association
   - Arthritis Foundation
   - National Coalition for Osteoporosis and Related Bone Disease
   - National Institute for Occupational Safety and Health
   - National Institute of Arthritis and Musculoskeletal and Skin Diseases
   - National Osteoporosis Foundation
   - Osteogenesis Imperfecta Foundation
   - The American Occupational Therapy Association, Inc.
   - The National Institute of Health Osteoporosis and Related Bone Disease, National Resource Center
   - Worker Health Chartbook 2004

TAKE-AWAY POINTS

1. Musculoskeletal disorders have a significant impact on health in the United States. Not only are individuals and their families affected, but also the workforce. As part of the chain reaction, the health and financial state of America is also impacted. Prevention has become a top priority as demonstrated through Healthy People 2010 and The Bone and Joint Decade

2000–2010. Both initiatives are a driving force to decrease the incidence of musculoskeletal injuries and increased self-management of musculoskeletal conditions.

2. Arthritis comes in a variety of forms and is the most common form of musculoskeletal disorder. The Centers for Disease Control and Prevention recognizes this disease as the most common cause of disability in the United States. "With $13 million in Fiscal Year 2008 (FY2008) funding, CDC is working with the Arthritis Foundation, the National Association of Chronic Disease Directors (NACDD), state arthritis program directors, and other partners to improve quality of life for adults with arthritis" (see http://www.cdc.gov/nccdphp/publications/aag/arthritis.htm).

3. Motivational interviewing is an effective form of counseling for people afflicted with musculoskeletal disorders. Issues of mobility, exercise, dietary intake of calcium and vitamin D, smoking cessation, and medication administration are among the many topics that can be the focus of an encounter with a patient diagnosed with a musculoskeletal disorder.

4. Nurses, among other things, are educators. With permission, we can educate our patients so they have the knowledge to make informed decisions. We must also respect the patient's desire to decline our offer to share information. It is important to fully assess what the patient knows so we are not offering information he or she already has. This can cause the patient to feel as though the nurse is superior and goes against the motivational interviewing concept of working in a partnership with the patient.

SUMMARY

Musculoskeletal disorders affect millions of Americans, and more are affected each day through a new diagnosis or injury. Although prevention will help to decrease the number of cases, we must also focus on the population already affected. We can promote self-management skills, provide education and counseling, and provide support for patients when they are ready to make a change. Additional research is needed to prove the effectiveness of motivational interviewing with musculoskeletal disorders. Ongoing utilization of the motivational interviewing tactics will provide useful information for further research.

REFERENCES

Arthritis Foundation. (2008). News from the arthritis foundation: Osteoarthritis fact sheet. Atlanta, GA: Arthritis Foundation.

Bergman, S. (2007). Public health perspective—How to improve the musculoskeletal health of the population. *Best Practice & Research Clinical Rheumatology, 21*(1), 191–204.

Elliott, R. (2008). Poor adherence to medication in adults with rheumatoid arthritis. *Disease Management Health Outcomes, 16*(1), 13–29.

Keefe, F., Lefebvre, J., Kerns, R., Rosenberg, R., Beaupre, P., Prochaska, J., Prochaska, J. O., & Caldwell, D. (2000). Understanding the adoption of arthritis self-management: Stages of change profiles among arthritis patients. *Pain, 87*(3), 303–313.

Koehn, C., & Esdaile, J. (2008). Patient education and self-management of musculo-skeletal diseases. *Best Practice and Research Clinical Rheumatology, 22*(3), 395–405.

National Center for Health Statistics. (2009). *Health, United States, 2008.* Hyattsville, MD: U.S. Department of Health and Human Services, Centers for Disease Control and Prevention, pages 9–17.

Rollnick, S., Miller, M., & Butler, C. (2008). *Motivational interviewing in health care: Helping patients change behavior.* New York: The Guilford Press.

Sarzi-Puttini, P., Buskila, D., Carrabba, M., Doria, A., & Atzeni, F. (2008). Treatment strategy in fibromyalgia syndrome: Where are we now? *Seminars in Arthritis & Rheumatism, 37,* 353–365.

Walsh, N., Brooks, P., Hazes, J., Walsh, R., Dreinhofer, K., Woolf, A., Akesson, K., & Lidgren, L. (2008). Standards of care for acute and chronic musculoskeletal pain: The bone and joint decade (2000–2010). *Archives of Physical Medicine and Rehabilitation, 89,* 1830–1845.

Yunus, M. (2007). Fibromyalgia and overlapping disorders: The unifying concept of central sensitivity syndromes. *Seminars in Arthritis & Rheumatism, 36,* 339–356.

CHAPTER 12

Motivational Interviewing in Mental Health Disorders

INTRODUCTION

Mental health disorders are significant in the United States. In 2004 the U.S. Census residential population estimated that 57.7 million people are afflicted with a mental health condition. Forty-five percent have at least two mental health diagnoses. These mental health disorders can range from mild to severe. Diagnosis is made based on the ***Diagnostic and Statistical Manual of Mental Disorders,* fourth edition** (see http://nimh.nih.gov/health/publications/the-numbers-count-mental-disorders-in-america/index.shtml). Because of the limited scope of this text, we look at disorders such as alcohol and drug abuse, depression, bipolar, anxiety, **obsessive-compulsive disorder**, eating disorders, and **attention deficit hyperactivity disorder**. There are a number of other disorders that could be mentioned, but they are demonstrated by irrational thinking, delusions, hallucinations, or paranoid thinking. This group of patients who are not institutionalized would likely require motivational interviewing interactions to take place with a family member.

Mood disorders encompass **major depressive disorder** (**MDD**), dysthymia, and bipolar disorder. Mood disorders as a group account for an estimated 20.9 million Americans over the age of 18. The average age at onset is 30 years. Depression is a common comorbid condition (see http://nimh.nih.gov/health/publications/the-numbers-count-mental-disorders-in-america/index.shtml). Mood disorders are often misunderstood. People suffering from these disorders live with a negative stigma that has only recently abated due to increased advertising and education of the population.

MDD and dysthymia are closely related. Dysthymia is a mild, chronic form of depression. MDD is an acute, more severe form of depression. Both forms are prevalent in America, with 14.8 million adults experiencing MDD each year. Dysthymia affects 3.3 million adults in any given year. The average age at onset for both forms of depression is in the early 30s. More women than men suffer from MDD. It was not noted which gender, if either, is more likely to be affected by dysthymia (see http://nimh.nih.gov/health/publications/the-numbers-count-mental-disorders-in-america/index.shtml).

Bipolar disorder, once termed manic-depressive disorder, swings between mania and depression. Bipolar disorder is diagnosed on average at age 25 years. An estimated 5.7 million American adults are affected in any given year. Different problems come with each end of the spectrum. When patients start moving into the manic phase, there is increased risk for suicide because they now have the energy to follow through with suicidal thoughts they may have experienced during depression (see http://nimh.nih.gov/health/publications/the-numbers-count-mental-disorders-in-america/index.shtml).

Although not a mental health disorder, suicide is a product of a mental health disorder. More than 90% of suicides occur in people who have a diagnosable mental health disorder. An estimated 32,439 suicides occurred in the United States in 2004. More women attempt suicide, but more men are successful and die by suicide. In 2006 there were 594,000 emergency room visits for self-inflicted injuries. Clearly, there is a need to improve these statistics (see http://www.cdc.gov/nchs/faststats/suicide.htm and http://nimh.nih.gov/health/publications/the-numbers-count-mental-disorders-in-america/index.shtml).

Obsessive-compulsive disorder begins in childhood but is often not diagnosed until an average age of 19. There are an estimated 2.2 million adults with obsessive-compulsive disorder in the United States in any given year. As with many mental health disorders there is a range of mild to severe forms. The mild forms often go undiagnosed and do not interfere with daily living. Some forms severely limit one's ability to accomplish daily tasks with ease (see http://nimh. nih.gov/health/publications/the-numbers-count-mental-disorders-in-america/ index.shtml).

Anxiety often goes hand in hand with depressive disorders. It can also be found with many chronic illnesses because there is a fear of the unknown, which triggers the anxiety. Anxiety can make it difficult to complete the simplest of tasks and can interfere with sleep, activities of daily living, and relationships. In 2006 the Centers for Disease Control and Prevention (CDC) reported that 11.3% of the population reported experiencing anxiety at some point in their lifetime. Common comorbidities include cardiovascular disease, diabetes, asthma, obesity, heavy drinking, smoking, and limited physical activity (see http://www.cdc.gov/Features/dsBRFSSDepressionAnxiety/).

Attention deficit hyperactivity disorder has become a growing problem in the United States. In 2007 the CDC reported approximately 4.5 million children between the ages of 3 and 17 years were diagnosed with attention deficit hyperactivity disorder. More boys than girls are diagnosed. This diagnosis brings many challenges to children's lives, such as social relationships, schooling, and overall emotional status. The impact on families is also significant (see http://www.cdc.gov/nchs/fastats/adhd.htm).

Eating disorders pose many challenges to patients, families, and healthcare providers. Between 2004 and 2006 there were about 32,000 hospital discharges each year with an eating disorder listed as one of the diagnoses. From 2003 to 2006 there was an average of 611,700 visits to physician offices and hospital outpatient and emergency rooms for eating disorders. In 2005 there were 56 deaths as a direct result of an eating disorder. There were another 78 deaths in which eating disorders contributed to the death but were not listed as the primary cause of death. Because eating disorders cause many other health problems that actually lead to death, the statistics are not as accurate as they could be. Most cases were patients less than 25 years of age (see http://www.cdc.gov/nchs/data/infosheets/infosheet_eatingbehaviors.htm).

Alcohol and drug abuse has been an ongoing problem in the United States. It affects young and old and does not discriminate among racial or financial backgrounds. In 2006 61% of adults drank alcohol in the past year and 20% had five or more drinks on at least one day. Approximately 75,000 deaths occur each year as a result of excessive alcohol intake. Forty-one percent of all motor vehicle accidents occur as a result of alcohol. It is alarming how alcohol also impacts the lives of our youth. The following statistics from 2007 give insight to this issue:

- 26% of high school students reported episodic heavy or binge drinking
- 11% of high school students reported drinking and driving over the previous 30 days
- 29% of high school students reported riding with someone who was drinking and driving

In 2006 there were 22,073 alcohol-related deaths, not including accidents or homicides. Alcohol severely affects the liver, and 13,050 alcoholic liver disease deaths occurred in 2006 (see http://www.cdc.gov/nchs/fastats/alcohol.htm and http://www.cdc.gov/HealthyYouth/alcoholdrug/).

Illegal drug use is another growing problem in the United States. Eighteen- to 25-year-olds have the highest use of illicit drugs. The CDC gathered data on people ages 12 years and older. Unfortunately, there are children 12 years old and even younger experimenting with or addicted to illegal drugs. Illegal drugs range from marijuana, cocaine, to heroin, and drug use also includes the nonmedical use of prescription or over-the-counter medications. In 2006, 8.3% of those older than 12 years of age had some form of illicit drug use over the past month. Six percent used marijuana over the past month. The most commonly used illegal drug in our younger population, the use of marijuana decreased from 27% to 20% from 1999 to 2007. Cocaine use increased from 2% in 1991 to 3% in 2007. Inhalant use was reported to be at 13% in 2007. Ecstasy, another illegal drug, was reported to be at 6% lifetime use in 2007. Methamphetamine use was at 4% in 2007. Heroin remained steady at 2% from 1999 to 2007. Hallucinogenic drug use was at 8% in 2007. There has been a decrease overall in illicit drug use. Interestingly, the use of prescription and over-the-counter drug use for recreation has increased. Prescription drugs were abused by 2.1 million teens in 2006. Statistics were not available for the use of over-the-counter medications (National Center for Health Statistics, 2009; seehttp://www.cdc.gov/HealthyYouth/alcoholdrug/).

Healthy People 2010 recognized the depth of the problem we have with mental health disorders. Focus areas were developed for mental health and mental disorders, in addition to substance abuse, which includes both drugs and alcohol. Prevention is necessary as we move toward a healthier nation. William Miller knew the difficulties of treating patients with addictions and developed motivational interviewing to improve treatment and potentially prevent recurrences. There has already been a decrease in the use of some substances for which there must be a variety of reasons. As we move forward and use the tools provided through motivational interviewing, our hope is to improve all of our statistics and create a healthier nation (see http://www.healthypeople.gov/About/ hpfact.htm).

CHALLENGES IN MENTAL HEALTH DISORDERS

The challenges in mental health care are endless. Mental health disorders often carry a negative stigma, and this prevents many from seeking care. Not only must they worry about what other people in their community might think, but they also must deal with their own family members and friends not understanding. Mental health disorders are complicated, and many people believe that we have power over our own thoughts and actions. To an extent this is true, but chemical malfunctions in the brain do occur and are difficult for those not experiencing it for themselves to comprehend.

Access to health care is limited. For those with insurance, coverage is limited to a certain number of visits. When those visits are utilized, patients either have to pay full payment for services or go without care. Many have no coverage at all. Services are also limited. Psychiatric care providers have waiting lists to be seen. This can be very frustrating for those suffering with symptoms that are not considered life threatening but are impairing function and decreasing quality of life.

Another challenge to managing mental health disorders is that they often coexist with physical disorders. Many healthcare providers focus on the physical issue first or may dismiss physical symptoms as part of their mental disorder. Depression, for one, often causes a variety of physical symptoms. When discussing with a general practitioner, it may be easier for them to assume it is related to the depressive disorder. Often, the first complaint of depression is followed up by ruling out physical causes. When physical and mental symptoms present together, it can be difficult to determine if one is causing the other. Too often, we do not see providers that have a good understanding of both physical and mental health.

A major challenge in mental health is the risk of suicide. Unnecessarily, lives are lost due to the strains of mental illness. Many are homeless and have lost their families and loved ones, their jobs, and their quality of life. Many feel hopeless, and the despair brings them to a point where they feel their only option is suicide.

In the area of addictions, the challenge lies in accepting there is a problem. Denial is common, and it is difficult to make behavior changes when there is no perceived problem. It is often repetitive, something people tend to fall back into when there are certain triggers. Each person has different triggers to self-medicate or get lost in a place they can create through the use of drugs and/or alcohol.

The **Substance Abuse & Mental Health Services Administration (SAMHSA)** recognizes the many challenges in our mental health system. The Federal Mental Health Action Agenda was created to "alter the form and function of the mental health service delivery system in this country to one that puts individuals–adults with mental illnesses, children with emotional disturbances, and family members–at its very core" (see http://samhsa.gov/Federalactionagenda/ NFC_FMHAA. aspx). The Federal Mental Health Action Agenda is detailed to specific actions to take and who is responsible for initiating the action. See Figure 12-1 for the goals of this initiative. This is just the first step in transforming our mental healthcare system. As we proceed with this initiative, some of these challenges will be reduced, if not eliminated.

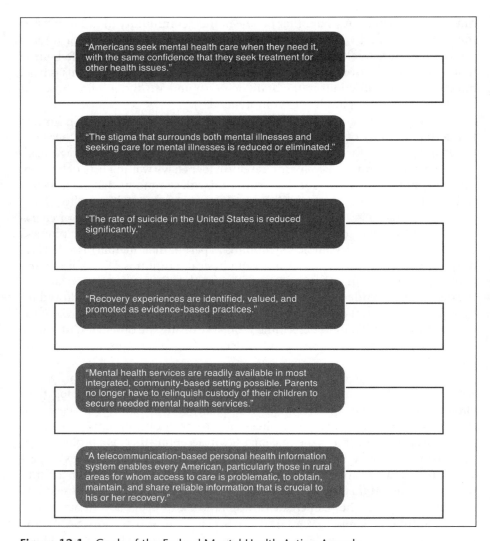

Figure 12-1 Goals of the Federal Mental Health Action Agenda

Source: http://www.samhsa.gov/Federalactionagenda/NFC_FMHAA.aspx

BENEFITS OF SELF-MANAGEMENT

The ability to self-manage a mental health disorder can provide the self-confidence needed to make changes and maintain changes. During a mental health crisis the goal is to help the patient become stable and to think and act in a rational manner. Self-management is not realistic during times of crisis. Once a patient can actively participate in self-care, it is important to support self-management. This builds their confidence and self-efficacy. Patients who lack self-efficacy are not likely to adhere to treatment recommendations. "People with mental illness who self-stigmatize tend to report little personal empowerment in terms of treatment so that participation in services is diminished. Hence, interventions that challenge self-stigma and facilitate empowerment are likely to improve adherence" (O'Donohue & Levensky, 2006, p. 388).

There is a strong focus on mental health promotion. The goal is to increase the sense of control over one's situation, build resiliency, and enhance one's ability to manage life around the mental health disorder. Often, what is offered through the mental health system is insufficient. Each individual patient is walking down his or her own personal path alone. No one can experience an exact replication of each patient's experience. What we can do as support persons is to help them enhance their experience (Young & Hayes, 2002). "It is perhaps an act of faith to accept that one is not responsible for the decisions made by another adult with whom one enters into a therapeutic contract, and that ultimately no-one can truly know what is 'best' for another person" (Kent, 2004, p. 41). For this reason it is essential to promote self-management.

Miller and Rollnick (2002) found that persons with addictions have a particularly hard time working through ambivalence. "People who are struggling with problem drinking, drug addiction, bulimia, or pathological gambling often recognize the risks, costs, and harm involved in their behavior. Yet for a variety of reasons they are also quite attached and attracted to the addictive behavior" (Miller & Rollnick, 2002, p. 14). Resolving this ambivalence is an important step to attaining self-control and improving self-management. Clients not actively involved in decision making are not likely to make lasting, effective changes, which can ultimately affect their future. Being involved in self-management places more responsibility on the patient, who is ultimately the one who knows what can realistically be accomplished and what is important to change (Wagner & McMahon, 2004).

There are some cases where self-management is not best and care should be dictated by the provider. This is an area of debate. Determining if a person is competent to make decisions becomes an ethical issue as well as a judgment call. One study examined the practice of patients with anorexia being forced into hospitalization with consequential forced feedings. Some debate that they are not mentally capable of making decisions about their health because of their distorted body image. Others would debate that alcoholics should all be forced into treatment because, ultimately, their life is at risk, too. This debate is beyond the scope of this text but needs to be mentioned because it adds to the complexity of managing mental health disorders (Thiels, 2008).

Ultimately, we know that being able to participate in one's own care increases the success of behavior change. Having a mental health disorder does not prevent one from being able to participate in one's own care. Self-management should be promoted despite disabilities or disparities. Increased confidence leads to motivation to improve areas that are holding us back from reaching our highest potential.

CASE STUDIES

The following case studies demonstrate useful tactics in motivational interviewing with patients who suffer from mental health disorders. In contrast, the case studies also show interactions that do not use motivational interviewing techniques.

Case Study 1

The patient has been suffering from anorexia. She has been in counseling for several years. She is coming in for follow-up.

Interaction Without Motivational Interviewing

> Nurse: Good morning. How are you doing today?
> Patient: I have been doing well.
> Nurse: So, you are maintaining your weight?
> Patient: I don't know for sure.
> Nurse: Do you feel your eating behaviors are under control?
> Patient: Yes, I guess so.
> Nurse: Have you been exercising?
> Patient: Yes.
> Nurse: How often do you exercise?
> Patient: A couple times a week, maybe.
> Nurse: What do you do for exercise?
> Patient: I run.
> Nurse: How about any forced vomiting?
> Patient: No, I never do that.
> Nurse: Is there any use of laxatives or diuretics?
> Patient: No.
> Nurse: So, it sounds like you are doing very well. Good for you.

Motivational Interviewing Interaction

> Nurse: Good morning. How are you doing?
> Patient: I'm doing well.

Nurse: I understand you are still in therapy. How is that going for you?

Patient: It's okay, I guess. Some days I leave there feeling pretty good about things and then other days I leave there feeling worse than when I walked in.

Nurse: Tell me more about that.

Patient: Well, there are times when I get caught up in the whole weight issue and I want to stop that. But when I go to therapy, sometimes she makes me come up with a plan to change and I just can't think of what I can do different. (Ambivalence)

Nurse: You feel torn between wanting to change and feeling too overwhelmed to make a plan for how you could go about that.

Patient: Yes. I don't even know where to start.

Nurse: Could you share with me a typical day for you?

Patient: Well, I usually get up pretty early and feel anxious, so I go for a run. When I get back, I have a small protein shake. I get ready for work, but when I look in the mirror, I get depressed because I see someone I don't even feel like I know.

Nurse: (silent)

Patient: I usually get through work without much problem. That's because I'm so busy. But after work, if I don't have anything planned, I have a hard time and feel anxious again, so I might go running. I usually come home, shower, eat a bowl of vegetables, and go to bed early.

Nurse: When busy or distracted, you do fine. But when you have a little free time, you get anxious. What are your thoughts about why you feel anxious?

Patient: It's like I fight with myself. I go through the arguments about the eating, the exercise, how I look, and it overwhelms me. I know I can't keep living like this, but I can't stop these thoughts.

Nurse: That must be a terrible feeling.

Patient: It is. That's why I run. I try to run away from the thoughts in my head.

Nurse: Have you had any thoughts about other ways to manage besides running?

Patient: Well, I know I should limit the exercise and I was thinking about doing some writing.

Nurse: What might you write about?

Patient: I have always wanted to write a book and I have so many ideas, but I just haven't taken the time to write anything down.

Nurse: You have a dream.

Patient: Yes, I guess you could call it that.

Nurse: What do you think prevents you from following through with that dream?

Patient: Fear.

Nurse: (silent)

Patient: I'm afraid I can't do it or that I will get too sick from the anorexia to finish it.

Nurse: You are afraid you might die as a result of the anorexia.

Patient: It is possible. I know that.

Nurse: You deserve to fulfill your dreams.

Patient: I do. I've never let anything stand in my way before. There's no reason to let the anorexia keep me from living my dream. (Change talk)

Nurse: I am confident that you will fulfill your dream once you set your mind to it.

Patient: Thank you.

Discussion

In the previous two scenarios the patient has an eating disorder that has not been well controlled for several years. In the first scenario the nurse asked direct questions that did not encourage the patient to expand on her answers. She gave the nurse limited information and likely what she thought the nurse wanted to hear. Patients with eating disorders can be manipulative and not completely honest when faced with such direct questioning. There was no time taken to build a rapport or gain trust, which is even more important when interacting with patients who have mental health disorders because trust is often an issue. This interaction was not successful at reaching the patient, eliciting information, or determining the patient's readiness for change.

In the second scenario the nurse builds a rapport and shows an interest in how the patient feels she is doing. Asking about a typical day allows the patient to share information that can give insight into the patient's barriers and needs for change. With guidance, the patient was able to find alternatives to replace negative behaviors. The nurse was supportive and voiced confidence in the patient. This in turn increases the patient's self-confidence. Motivational interviewing is an effective tool to help patients evaluate their situation and find possible solutions (Rollnick, Miller, & Butler, 2008).

Case Study 2

The patient is suffering from depression and is having suicidal thoughts.

Interaction Without Motivational Interviewing

Nurse: Good morning. How are you today?

Patient: I can't keep going. I just want to end it all.

Nurse: Tell me what is going on.

Patient: I just don't have the strength to keep living. I lost my job. My relationship is suffering, and I see no solutions.

Nurse: You obviously have a lot going on. Have you talked to your counselor or psychiatrist?

Patient: No.

Nurse: I would recommend you call your counselor and see if you can get an appointment.

Patient: Okay.

Nurse: Now do you have anything I can help you with today?

Patient: No, I guess not.

Motivational Interviewing Interaction

Nurse: Good morning. How are you?

Patient: I can't take it anymore. I just can't keep going.

Nurse: You are feeling hopeless.

Patient: Yes, I am. I lost my job. My relationship is ending. And I feel like I'm falling apart.

Nurse: You have a lot on your plate right now.

Patient: You can say that again.

Nurse: I would like to ask if you are feeling as though you might harm yourself right now.

Patient: I've thought about it. I'll be honest with you. I haven't done anything, but I have thought about it.

Nurse: You realized your life is worth living.

Patient: No. My life is a mess and I feel so alone.

Nurse: So, what is keeping you from following through with it?

Patient: I don't really want to die.

Nurse: Life is worth living. You are worthwhile.

Patient: I don't know. It just hurts so badly inside that I don't want to keep feeling this way, but at the same time I don't want to kill myself. (Ambivalence)

Nurse: It's like you have two demons inside you battling.

Patient: It kind of feels that way.

Nurse: Tell me about a time you might have felt this way before.

Patient: Oh, that was about 10 years ago. I got really depressed after I graduated from college. I think I was just overwhelmed with the future and all the responsibilities.

Nurse: What got you through that time?

Patient: I started writing in a journal.

Nurse: (silent)

Patient: I would write about how I was feeling and then when I looked back at what I wrote, I realized how irrational I was being. Even now, I know my thoughts are irrational. Losing a job and a relationship is not worth dying for.

Nurse: You found clarity in your writing.

Patient: Yes, I did. I'm going to get a journal and try that again.

Nurse: That sounds like a good plan. I would love to hear how it is going. Would you like to come back next week?

Patient: Sure.

Discussion

In the previous two scenarios the patient is suffering from depression and is clearly at risk to harm herself. In the first scenario the nurse does not address the issues but instead tries to pass the problem onto the counselor. A patient who is in this situation needs prompt attention. This is a situation that nurses can be presented with and need to be prepared to address it. There is also a legal obligation to ensure the safety of our patients, and this patient is at risk.

In the second scenario the nurse encouraged the patient to openly discuss her feelings about suicide and explore other options. By actively listening, offering reflections, and asking open-ended questions the nurse and patient formed a therapeutic relationship. The nurse encouraged the patient to look back to a similar situation and evaluate what was effective in the past. The patient decided that what worked in a similar situation was worth trying again. The patient left the encounter feeling hope. When motivational interviewing is used properly, the patient should leave the encounter feeling hopeful, rejuvenated, energized, and motivated. The nurse did not tell the patient what to do but helped her to find the solution that she believed would work best for her.

Case Study 3

The patient is a recovering alcoholic who has returned to drinking.

Interaction Without Motivational Interviewing

Nurse: Good morning. How have you been?

Patient: I'm sure you already know that I've been drinking again.

Nurse: Yes, I did know that. You had worked hard to stop drinking.

Patient: I know, but I just don't care anymore.

Nurse: I know that we have talked about all the possible negative consequences of drinking alcohol. Do we need to talk about that again?

Patient: No. I know all that and don't want to hear it again.

Nurse: So, you know all the negative aspects of drinking. Why do you keep going back?

Patient: I don't know. I guess it comforts me. And no matter what you say, it's not going to change.

Nurse: Maybe you don't want to talk about it right now. We can talk again next week.

Patient: Whatever. I don't think much is going to change between now and then.

Nurse: Well, do your best to try staying away from the alcohol. You were able to do it before and I'm sure you can do it again.

Patient: We'll see.

Motivational Interviewing Interaction

Nurse: Good morning. How are you?

Patient: I'm sure you already know that I am drinking again.

Nurse: You have had an interesting journey. What are your thoughts about what brought you here today?

Patient: Well, I had been good. I hadn't been drinking in a year. Then my father got sick and I had him come stay with me and my family so we could help him out.

Nurse: (silent)

Patient: It started up the same old thing. He tells me how stupid and worthless I am and that I'm nothing but a drunk.

Nurse: You believe him when he tells you those things.

Patient: I try not to, but it's hard. I thought he would be proud of me and how far I came. But instead he tells me what a loser I am. I might as well be what he thinks I already am. (Resistance)

Nurse: You allowed your father to tear you down.

Patient: I did allow it, didn't I? I didn't think of it that way.

Nurse: A parent is supposed to build you up, not tear you down.

Patient: My father wouldn't know how to build me up. But I also don't have to allow him to tear me down anymore. (Ambivalence)

Nurse: That is true. You have choices.

Patient: It's hard to change something that has been happening for years and years.

Nurse: It is difficult, but nothing is impossible.

Patient: You are right. I don't have to live like this. I don't have to believe what my father says. I can believe in myself.

Nurse: You know you can do this. You were already there.

Patient: You know, I am going to stop drinking. I don't like drinking anymore. (Change talk)

Nurse: Many things trigger people to drink. Having a plan to deal with those triggers can be helpful. What are your thoughts about that?

Patient: Do you mean how will I deal with my father?

Nurse: Any situation that triggers you to want to drink.

Patient: Well, for the sake of my health, I'm going to avoid situations where my father can put me down. If he starts, I will leave. My AA sponsor said I could call him anytime. That might be a good time to do that.

Nurse: So, there are some ways for you to get back on track and avoid another relapse.

Patient: Yes, I guess there are.

Nurse: I like to see my patients who have relapsed about once a week. How does that sound for you?

Patient: I can do that.

Discussion

In the previous two scenarios the patient is an alcoholic who has relapsed. The first scenario is not effective in areas of eliciting information to determine the source of the problem, assessing readiness, or properly dealing with patient resistance. The nurse does not form a therapeutic relationship. The nurse makes the assumption that the patient will come back in a week. By asking "why do you keep going back" implies the patient is making a conscious, rational decision. The nurse does not ask enough open-ended questions to elicit information. The patient was resistant, and this should have told the nurse to evaluate her words, body language, and overall approach to the patient. The nurse may have had some values that were being projected and could have been seen to act superior to the patient. This was not a partnership.

In the second scenario motivational interviewing was used. This was a more productive encounter. The nurse expressed concern, was nonjudgmental, and worked with the patient to find what needed to change and methods of coping with obstacles to maintaining sobriety. The nurse recognizes this is a challenging issue and validates the patient's feelings that it is a struggle to get and stay sober. The patient was not criticized. He was able to explore the situation openly with the nurse and find a way to make sobriety work for him. These are the encounters for which motivational interviewing was created.

PRACTICE TOOLS (FIGURE 12-2)

1. When trying to understand about the patient's lifestyle, barriers, and successes, ask the patient to describe a typical day. This is an alternative way to asking close-ended questions. By using this technique you can unearth valuable information. The following potential information could be revealed:

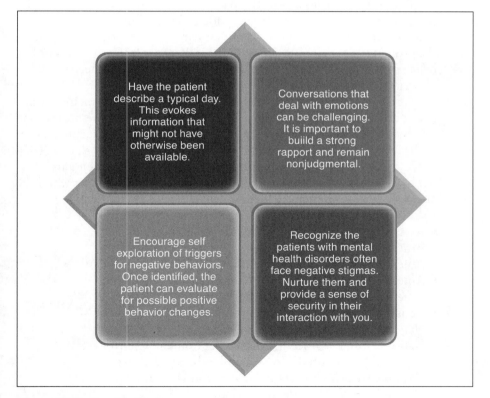

Figure 12-2   Practice Tools

- What is the daily routine?
- Are they eating and getting routine exercise?
- How do they spend their time?
- What barriers are perceived?
- What stressors do they have?
- What is working well for them?
- Are there successes that deserve praise?

2. Expect conversations to be difficult. Patients are often dealing with their innermost emotions, and this is very challenging for the patient to share. A strong rapport must be established. Many times it may be difficult for them to identify their emotions, stressors, and barriers to change. The nurse can play an important role in helping the patient increase self-awareness and objectively evaluate the positive and negative aspects of a situation.

3. Inquire about triggers for negative behaviors. This may be difficult to determine but will at least help the patient to become more aware of the possible triggers. We all have triggers. Identifying them can be a challenge and requires self-exploration. The nurse can support the patient as he or she evaluates a personal situation to see if there are triggers for his or her behaviors. Once identified, the patient can then proceed to determine appropriate changes that can be made for improvement.

4. The nurse must have a strong sense of self-awareness. Many mental health disorders carry a negative stigma. If the patient suspects the nurse to be anything but nonjudgmental, the patient will not feel the trust necessary to delve into his or her issues. Patients often carry guilt and shame. They need to feel safe and secure in their interactions to share their story. Listen to their story. Do not pass judgment. Accept the patient for who they are and what issues they are facing.

5. Use available resources:
   - American Academy of Addiction Psychiatry
   - American Academy of Child and Adolescent Psychiatry
   - American Psychiatric Association
   - American Psychiatric Nurses Association
   - American Psychological Association
   - Centers for Disease Control and Prevention
   - National Alliance on Mental Illness
   - National Center for Injury and Prevention and Control
   - **National Center on Addiction and Substance Abuse**
   - National Clearinghouse for Alcohol and Drug Information
   - National Eating Disorders Association
   - National Institute of Mental Health

- National Institute on Alcohol Abuse and Alcoholism
- National Institute on Drug Abuse
- Substance Abuse and Mental Health Services Administration

TAKE-AWAY POINTS

1. Mental health disorders have a significant impact on the health of our nation. When mild, patients can lead a normally productive life. When severe, patients can be completely debilitated, unable to work or live independently. This has an effect on families, employers, and any social supports. In addition to Healthy People 2010, the SAMHSA has developed a plan to improve our mental healthcare system.
2. Patients with mental health disorders live with guilt and shame. With the use of motivational interviewing these patients can build their self-confidence and become more self-efficacious. Our goal is to support these patients in their self-management.
3. Motivational interviewing has long been known to be effective in addictions counseling. This set of disorders is the cornerstone on which motivational interviewing was created and built to be a strong force in the area of behavior change. Motivational interviewing has also been found to be effective in many areas of health care. As nurses, we are at the forefront of this movement.
4. Every interaction has numerous possibilities. The way we communicate with our patients can significantly impact the outcome. As a caring profession, nurses have the ability to reach millions. Each negative behavior that we can help change to positive can have an impact on the health of our entire nation.

SUMMARY

Millions of Americans suffer from one, if not more than one, mental health disorder. Nurses are often in the position to help the patients of this population. Every interaction is important. Healthy People 2010 strives to decrease the nation's incidence of mental health disabilities and substance abuse. Motivational interviewing has had a positive impact on this population. As we move toward the future, this creative method of health promotion will be the basis from which we promote behavior change.

REFERENCES

Kent, R. (2004). Trust me, I'm a client–Embracing motivational interviewing. *Drugs and Alcohol Today,* 4(2), 37–42.

Miller, W., & Rollnick, S. (2002). Motivational interviewing: Preparing people for change, 2nd ed. New York: The Guilford Press.

National Center for Health Statistics. (2009). *Health, United States, 2008.* Hyattsville, MD: U.S. Department of Health and Human Services, Centers for Disease Control and Prevention, pages 9–17.

O'Donohue, W., & Levensky, E. (2006). *Promoting treatment adherence: A practical handbook for healthcare providers.* Thousand Oaks, CA: Sage Publications.

Rollnick, S., Miller, W., & Butler, C. (2008). *Motivational interviewing in health care: Helping patients change behavior.* New York: The Guilford Press.

Thiels, C. (2008). Forced treatment of patients with anorexia. *Current Opinion in Psychiatry, 21*(5), 495–498.

Wagner, C., & McMahon, B. (2004). Motivational interviewing and rehabilitation counseling practice. *Rehabilitation Counseling Bulletin, 47*(3), 152–161.

Young, L., & Hayes, V. (2002). *Transforming health promotion practice: Concepts, issues, and applications.* Philadelphia: F.A. Davis.

CHAPTER 13

Motivational Interviewing in Pulmonary Disorders

OBJECTIVES

After completing this chapter, the reader will be able to

1. Identify three pulmonary disorders that have a negative impact on health in the United States.
2. Discuss three challenges in managing pulmonary health.
3. List three benefits of self-management in pulmonary health.
4. Report how motivational interviewing can be used effectively in managing pulmonary health.
5. Create three metaphors that could be useful in an encounter with a patient who is struggling with ambivalence.

KEY TERMS

Cystic fibrosis (CF)
Chronic obstructive pulmonary disease (COPD)
Influenza-like illness
Influenza A (H_1) (seasonal influenza)
Influenza A (H_3) (seasonal influenza)
Influenza B (seasonal influenza)
National Asthma Control Program

National Asthma Education and Prevention Program
National Center for Environmental Health
Novel influenza A (H_1N_1) (swine flu)
Respiratory syncytial virus
Society for Public Health Education
World Health Organization

INTRODUCTION

Pulmonary disorders have a significant role in health in the United States. There are a variety of disorders that range from mild and acute to chronic and severe and are of a genetic source or acquired. Here we look at the most common chronic pulmonary disorders, such as asthma, **chronic obstructive pulmonary** disease (COPD), and cystic fibrosis (CF), and acute disorders, such as influenza and respiratory syncytial virus. Although smoking is a major contributing factor to many respiratory disorders, it is covered in Chapter 14.

COPD encompasses the disorders of chronic bronchitis and emphysema. Chronic bronchitis afflicted 7.6 million Americans in 2006. Seven hundred forty people died from chronic bronchitis that year. In 2006, 3.7 million people were found to have ever been diagnosed with emphysema, 12,551 deaths from emphysema occurred, and 107,679 deaths occurred from other chronic lower respiratory diseases (not including asthma) (see http://www.cdc.gov/nchs/fastats/copd.htm).

CF is a genetic disease of chronic nature that affects both the pulmonary and gastrointestinal systems. In the pulmonary system secretions are very thick and sticky and can lead to life-threatening lung infections. There are approximately 1,000 new cases of CF each year, with greater than 70% diagnosed by age 2. In the 1950s children with CF rarely lived to attend elementary school. Now the average survival age is greater than 37 years. Mandatory prenatal testing now allows for earlier diagnosis and treatment, which has contributed to this lengthened life expectancy (see http://www.cff.org/AboutCF/index.cfm?dspPrintReady=Y).

Asthma has had a tremendous impact on health in the United States. The most recent data state that 16.2 million American adults and 6.7 million American children have asthma. There are approximately 10.6 million physician visits a year for asthma-related illness. In 2006 inpatient hospitalizations for first-time diagnosis was 444,000 and 3,613 deaths were related to asthma (see http://www.cdc.gov/nchs/FASTATS/asthma.htm). In 2001 the Society for Public Health Education published the "Resolution on Reducing the Impact of Asthma." This report stated that asthma was the leading cause of school absences for a chronic illness. Over 10 million school days were missed per year. The financial impact of asthma in 2000 was noted to be an estimated annual cost of 12.7 billion dollars. Clearly, there is work to be done to improve asthma statistics (see http://www.sophe.org/public/nhew/asthma/asthmres.html).

In 2007 the Centers for Disease Control and Prevention (CDC) published the report "National Surveillance for Asthma—United States, 1980–2004." This report provided more detailed information about the negative impact asthma has on U.S. health. The CDC found a need to take a public health approach to dealing with this chronic disease because there are ways to reduce the occurrence of exacerbations. The following results were published in this report (see http://www.cdc.gov/mmwr/preview/mmwrhtml/ss5608a1.htm):

- In 2001–2003 there were 20 million persons in the United States with asthma.
- 8.5% of children and 6.7% of adults were afflicted.

- In childhood, more males were affected.
- In adulthood, more females were affected.
- People with low family income are most affected.
- There were an average 11.6 million people with one asthma attack during the previous 12 months, with an average 11 million per year between 1997 and 2004.
- There were an average 12.3 million physician visits per year between 2001 and 2003.
- Between 2001 and 2003 there were an average 1.8 million emergency room visits due to asthma, with 1.1 million being in the adult population and 696,900 being in the pediatric population.
- There was an average of 4,210 deaths related to asthma annually between 2001 and 2003.
- 50% of the deaths were people aged 65 or older and about 200 deaths in children younger than 18.

Respiratory syncytial virus causes bronchiolitis and pneumonia in children younger than 1 year of age. There are 75,000 to 125,000 children hospitalized because of respiratory syncytial virus each year. What is interesting is that most children are infected by this virus by the age of 2, but only a small percentage of these children develop a severe enough form to be hospitalized. Adults who are immunocompromised and adults over the age of 65 are also at risk to develop a severe form of this disease. Outbreaks of respiratory syncytial virus tend to occur between the months of November and April in the United States. Synagis is given to premature infants to protect against this virus, and there is no specific treatment (see http://cdc/gov/rsv/about/faq.html).

Influenza has been a challenging respiratory virus to manage. New immunizations are created for each flu season, but it is difficult to predict what strains are going to be most prevalent. In 2006 there were 849 deaths due to influenza. Data on immunizations received are only available in adults 65 years and older. Approximately 64% of adults received the influenza vaccine in 2006 (see http://www.cdc.gov/nchs/fastats/flu.htm).

The CDC provides a weekly summary of influenza statistics nationwide (see http://www.cdc.gov/flu/weekly). Seasonal influenza contributes to acute illness every year. This year the identification of novel influenza A (H_1N_1), or swine flu, has presented another risk to health in the United States. The information discussed in this section is from the week 27 report(July 5–11, 2009). There were 1,278 positive influenza tests. Almost 100% of these were novel influenza A (H_1N_1). There were nine states with widespread influenza activity. **Influenza A (H_1), influenza A (H_3),** and **influenza B** viruses have been documented throughout the 2008–2009 season. Statistics up to July 17, 2009 are as follows:

- 40,617 confirmed and probable infections with novel influenza A (H_1N_1)
- 211 deaths were identified by the CDC (ages 0–4 = 7 deaths; ages 5–24 = 43 deaths; ages 25–49 = 101 deaths; ages 50–64 = 66 deaths; 65 and older = 23 deaths; there were 22 deaths of unknown age)

Since October 1, 2008 the CDC identified 1,817 season influenza viruses and 233 **novel influenza A (H_1N_1)** viruses. During week 27, 6.5% of all deaths reported were due to pneumonia and influenza. The epidemic threshold is 6.6%. Since September 28, 2008 the CDC had received reports of pediatric deaths related to influenza, with 23 of those being novel influenza A (H_1N_1). During week 27 (July 5–11, 2009), about 1.3% of outpatient visits were for **influenza-like illness**. On June 11, 2009, the **World Health Organization** declared a global pandemic of novel influenza A (H_1N_1). There had been more than 70 countries affected with ongoing outbreaks. These data are invaluable to help us understand the effect that influenza has on our health. There is an obvious need to focus on prevention (see http://www.cdc.gov/flu/weekly and http://www.cdc.gov/h1n1flu/).

Healthy People 2010 focuses on environmental health and respiratory diseases as 2 of the 28 major focus areas. There are several objectives developed specifically for asthma, with the following goals:

- Reduce asthma-related deaths
- Reduce asthma-related hospitalizations
- Reduce emergency room visits for asthma
- Reduce activity limitations related to asthma
- Reduce the number of missed school and workdays related to asthma
- Increase asthma patient education
- Increase the number of patients with asthma who receive care according to the **National Asthma Education and Prevention Program**
- Establish an asthma surveillance program in at least 25 states

In 1999 the **National Asthma Control Program** was created by the **National Center for Environmental Health** to support the goals set forth by Healthy People 2010. Funding was provided to implement asthma interventions geared toward accomplishing these goals. As nurses, our role is to participate in these programs when available and to provide appropriate patient education and promote behavior change to assist in accomplishing these goals (see http://www.healthypeople.gov/About/hpfact.htm and http://www.cdc.gov/mmwr/preview/mmwrhtml/ss5608a1.htm).

CHALLENGES IN MANAGING PULMONARY DISORDERS

There are many challenges in managing disorders of the pulmonary system. One problem is preventing and controlling the acute viral infections. Many efforts are made to prevent illness, such as influenza and pneumonia, by use of vaccines. National campaigns that promote frequent hand washing and other tactics to decrease the spread of illness offer some protection. Despite these measures there are many office and emergency room visits and missed days at school and work due to respiratory illness. Review of protective tactics should be performed with our patients. As we have seen with diseases such as the swine flu, it is difficult to control the transmission of these acute illnesses, and they can easily reach pandemic proportions. Prevention can be difficult, yet it is one of the most important factors in decreasing the incidence of these diseases.

The treatment regimens for chronic pulmonary disorders can be complicated and difficult to maintain a routine. Cystic fibrosis requires many respiratory treatments and chest physiotherapy. This can be very time consuming and costly yet life saving. Patients and parents of young patients must have dedication to these therapies to decrease the risk of respiratory complications. Complications result in additional missed school and workdays and increased healthcare costs if resulting in hospitalization. Education about these therapies is necessary. Encouraging and supporting self-management is important for nurses to remember in each encounter.

Nonadherence to treatment regimens of asthma is also prevalent. There are many identified reasons for this. Lack of understanding about symptoms of asthma is one contributing factor. Many people also believe that when they feel well, there is no need for treatment. Preventive medication is very important in asthma management. Sometimes the provider does not prescribe adequate therapy to control symptoms (Elder & Mellon, 2008). The World Health Organization identifies the following as reasons for nonadherence to asthma medication treatment (Elliott, 2006):

- Fear of adverse effects of medication
- Fear of addiction
- Belief that medication is not effective or not needed
- Stigmatization
- Inconvenience
- Costs
- Dislike of provider; distrust of medical establishment
- Difficulty administering medication
- Interferes with life
- Division of responsibility between child and caregiver

Another challenge in managing pulmonary disorders is the limitations it places on a person's activity level. These patients are in a difficult situation when they know activity is important for their health yet it is limited by their health. They find it hard to prevent situations, such as an asthma exacerbation, and recovery can be made difficult due to the decreased activity. The risk of developing pneumonia increases with decreased activity. Ultimately, these patients struggle with the inconsistent activity and unpredictable exacerbations of symptoms. This can lead to other issues, such as depression and anxiety.

In diseases such as asthma, people of low income are more at risk. This poses many challenges in regards to access to health care, ability to obtain treatment due to financial constraints, transportation to receive health care, and missed work in an already strained financial situation. Although support has become more readily available, it can still be challenging to reach all people who are suffering from these afflictions.

Asthma may not be properly treated due to lack of diagnosis. Children have missed 22 million school days per year on account of acute upper respiratory infections. Recurrent respiratory illnesses could be caused by underlying asthma. Increased awareness of this fact can help practitioners to consider this when evaluating these children. Proper treatment of asthma can decrease the risk of these acute illnesses (Wingrove, 2009).

BENEFITS OF SELF-MANAGEMENT

When patients manage symptoms of their pulmonary disorders safely and effectively at home, they can significantly decrease the number of visits to physician offices and emergency rooms. Ultimately, it decreases the number of healthcare dollars used to manage the complications of these disorders. Being comfortable managing one's own illness increases the patient's self-confidence and motivation to demonstrate positive health behaviors.

The CDC recommends self-management of asthma for a couple reasons. Evidence has proven self-management to be effective in improving outcomes of chronic asthma. Also, there are many aspects of asthma management that can be prevented with proper self-management. Tasks, such as medication administration, monitoring symptoms with appropriate follow-up with the healthcare provider, and identification and avoidance of asthma triggers can be accomplished by the asthma patient. Self-management education is an important part of treatment. As we move toward attaining Healthy People 2010 goals, more self-management education is being provided. Motivational interviewing has been found to be effective in promoting positive behaviors in asthma management (Rubak, Sandboek, Lauritzen, & Christensen, 2005; see http://www.cdc.gov/mmwr/preview/mmwrhtml/mm5635a4.htm).

"Research has shown that self-efficacy beliefs are related to whether the person will attempt to perform a task and to how long he or she will persevere" (Bartholomew, Parcel, Swank, & Czyzewski, 1993, p. 1524). Just starting with positive behaviors is not enough. The patient must follow through with the regimen. This can be difficult for many reasons, as previously reported. As nurses, we must not only provide appropriate education, but we must help our patients to change perspectives and possibly habitual negative behaviors. Motivational interviewing can be used to help us provide the support our patients need. People who believe in themselves accomplish more, let fewer things get in the way of accomplishing their goals, and have an increased intrinsic motivation. Ongoing support for even those successful with self-management is important. Through the use of motivational interviewing, we can offer that support.

The path to improved health is long and can have many mountains and valleys. It is not an easy path. Any steps we can take to help patients decrease the risk factors for pulmonary disorders or decrease the triggers for exacerbations of existing pulmonary disorders will impact the health of our entire nation, as well as increase the quality of life for those suffering with these disorders.

CASE STUDIES

The following case studies look at nurse–patient interactions and compare nonmotivational interviewing and motivational interviewing styles of communication. All are patients diagnosed with a pulmonary disorder who could benefit from some positive behavior changes.

Case Study 1

The patient is a 4-year-old child with CF. The parent is struggling with administering his treatments on time every day.

Interaction Without Motivational Interviewing

Nurse: Good morning. How are you doing, today?

Parent: I'm good. How are you?

Nurse: I'm good, thanks. I see here that Hunter has had some respiratory problems lately. What's been going on?

Parent: I don't know. He just keeps getting worse.

Nurse: Are you giving him his treatments?

Parent: Well, I try to, but it's hard to stay on schedule with him.

Nurse: It is very important that he receives every treatment.

Parent: I know it is. I try, but you can't imagine what I go through to give him his treatments.

Nurse: I'm sure it must be difficult. Let's develop a plan for how you will get his treatments to him on time. It is important to stay on schedule.

Parent: Again, I know that. I'm doing the best I can.

Motivational Interviewing Interaction

Nurse: Good morning. How are you doing, today?

Parent: I'm good. How are you?

Nurse: I'm good, thanks. I see here that Hunter has had some respiratory problems lately. What are your thoughts about that?

Parent: I feel terrible. I hate to see him going through this.

Nurse: I'm sure you do. I can only imagine.

Parent: I feel so guilty that I could have prevented some of this.

Nurse: What makes you feel that way?

Parent: I try to keep him on schedule with his treatments, but it is so difficult. (Resistance)

Nurse: Tell me about the challenges you are facing.

Parent: Well, you know how active a 4-year-old can be. It is so hard to tame him down to do a treatment. I feel like I spend my entire day chasing him around just to give him his treatment. I get nothing else done.

Nurse: That must be very frustrating.

Parent: It is. But I also know that it makes it even harder on him. He can't enjoy his activities if I am running around yelling at him.

Nurse: So, neither one of you are able to enjoy your day if you have to spend every moment focused on the treatments.

Parent: No. So, I have skipped some treatments just so we can have some peace in our day. (Ambivalence)

Nurse: And you feel that those missed treatments have contributed to the recent illnesses.

Parent: Yes, I do. How do other parents do it?

Nurse: I'm sure there are numerous ways that families manage. What thoughts have you had about solutions?

Parent: I have thought about writing out a sort of schedule that might work. I just haven't had the time. (Change talk)

Nurse: Would you like to take a little time and sketch something out with me?

Parent: Sure. If there is any way you can help me find solutions to this problem, I would appreciate it.

Nurse: Tell me about how you envision your successful day.

Parent: Well, we would get up and everything would be all set up and ready to go. That way it's not a whole production just building up to it all. I guess I could do his chest therapy first. While he's doing that, I could get his breakfast and medication ready. That might make the morning go a little smoother.

Nurse: That sounds like a good start. You want to maybe have some time in the evening to get things set up so you can start your day in a more positive way.

Parent: That's right. I think that alone could make a huge difference.

Nurse: (silent)

Parent: I think once the morning rush is over, he can go play while I get the next round of treatments ready. I would love to be able to start dinner while I'm making lunch. Then right before lunch, I'll let him watch television while he gets his chest therapy. And then do the lunch routine.

Nurse: It sounds like you know what to do and you have some great ideas.

Parent: I think it can work. I can try to do the dinner routine about the same. This can definitely work. I'll get set up for the next morning when he goes to bed. I don't think I'll be so exhausted at the end of the day if I'm not spending it running after him and fighting with him to do his treatments.

Nurse: You really want the therapy routine to improve. I'm confident that once you find a system that works for you, you will have no problem sticking to it.

Discussion

In the previous two scenarios the nurse had an interaction with the parent of a 4-year-old child with CF. The problem the parent was experiencing was giving the respiratory treatments on schedule and he was missing treatments that are vital to preventing complications. In the first scenario the parent tried to discuss problems she was having with the treatment schedule and administration of therapies to her child. The nurse kept putting emphasis on how important it was to administer the treatments on schedule, instead of taking the time to explore the barriers the parent was struggling with. The nurse did not offer empathy, did not attempt to elicit information from the parent, and did not explore other options with the parent but evoked a sense that she was superior to the parent. This was not an effective therapeutic interaction as it did not promote improved self-management skills, allow the patient exploration of barriers, or encourage changes in behavior.

In the second scenario the nurse allows the parent to talk about what she felt the problems were that contributed to an increase in respiratory illnesses. The parent felt comfortable sharing her concerns. The parent came up with the solution on her own, with gentle guidance from the nurse. The parent was able to develop a plan for a more effective routine in administering the child's therapies. By asking the parent what she envisioned for a positive experience, the nurse was able to elicit additional information that might not otherwise been shared. The use of motivational interviewing shaped this into a successful and therapeutic communication between the nurse and the parent.

Case Study 2

The patient is a 16-year-old with asthma. She does not want to take her medication because she doesn't want her friends to think she is sick.

Interaction Without Motivational Interviewing

> Nurse: Good morning. How are you?
>
> Patient: I'm fine.
>
> Nurse: I see at the last visit you weren't taking your medication as prescribed. Are you taking your medication like you are supposed to?
>
> Patient: Sometimes.
>
> Nurse: How often would you say you are taking it?
>
> Patient: I take it before school, at bedtime, and sometimes after school, if I come right home.
>
> Nurse: And you are supposed to take it when?
>
> Patient: I'm supposed to take the short- and long-acting inhalers in the morning, the short acting before gym or soccer and then the long acting at bedtime and the short acting only if I really need it before bed.
>
> Nurse: So, you really just need to make sure you start taking your short-acting inhaler before gym and sports.
>
> Patient: Those are the ones I tend to miss.
>
> Nurse: Okay, so you can try to take it during those times and that should help.
>
> Patient: Okay.

Motivational Interviewing Interaction

> Nurse: Good morning. How are you?
>
> Patient: I'm okay.
>
> Nurse: What does okay mean for you?
>
> Patient: I mean I'm feeling pretty good.
>
> Nurse: Tell me about your asthma symptoms.

Patient: I usually feel pretty good, but I have noticed I get short of breath near the end of gym class and soccer practice or games.

Nurse: (silent)

Patient: I get this sort of tightness around my chest. It feels hard to take in a deep breath.

Nurse: That must be frightening. What helps make you feel better?

Patient: I just sit and rest for a few minutes.

Nurse: You take it easy and stop exercising until you can breathe easier.

Patient: Yes. It's hard because I want to get back in the game, but I end up sitting out because of it.

Nurse: Let me understand. You feel pretty good, except when you have any exercise. Then you get short of breath and have to rest.

Patient: That's right.

Nurse: Many people with asthma find they need additional medication to help get through exercise. What have you found helps you?

Patient: Well, it probably would help if I took the short-acting inhaler beforehand. (Ambivalence)

Nurse: (silent)

Patient: I just hate to do that. It's so hard to have to explain my asthma to everyone. And if I take time to use my inhaler, they all start asking questions and I feel like I'm a freak. (Resistance)

Nurse: You are concerned about the other kids making a big deal over your asthma, and it makes you feel different from them.

Patient: I am different from them.

Nurse: We are all different in some way. People get picked on for wearing glasses so they can see, having to carry epinephrine in case of a bee sting so they don't have an allergic reaction, or wearing an insulin pump, the lifeline for people with diabetes.

Patient: I never thought of it that way. I guess I'm not any different from some of them.

Nurse: It's not easy being different, but it gets easier when we realize we are not alone.

Patient: At least I don't have to have attention on my asthma all the time. I only have to worry about it when I'm exercising. (Change talk)

Nurse: You feel taking the medication before exercising may help solve your problem.

Patient: Yes, it probably would.

Nurse: I'm confident you will find a way to make it work for you so that you can be out on the soccer field more.

Patient: I hope so.

Discussion

In the previous two scenarios the nurse was working with an adolescent who is not adhering to her treatment regimen. In the first scenario the nurse did not inquire about perceived barriers. Without that information the discussion about improving self-management cannot be effective. The nurse did not assess how well the patient's asthma is controlled. This patient could be symptom free and changes may not be necessary at this time, or the asthma may be severe and persistent, requiring significant changes to improve symptoms. The nurse cannot possibly know what the patient needs to improve if she doesn't have any information. The first task a nurse should always complete is an assessment.

In the second scenario the nurse let the patient examine what the problem was and supported her as she searched for a solution. The nurse respectfully offered other perspectives to the patient's feelings of being different from her classmates and teammates. The nurse took time to summarize what she had heard, to ensure she had a good understanding of what the patient was describing as an issue for her. This also gave evidence that the nurse was actively listening to what the patient was saying. This tactic helps to build trust, a necessary component to therapeutic communication. The patient felt more comfortable discussing how she was really feeling. By using motivational interviewing, the conversation became one of the patient working toward behavior change. The nurse and patient worked as a team versus the nurse being in charge and the patient sitting idly by. The second scenario demonstrated the nurse and patient working together to face the obstacles that are presented in managing a chronic illness.

Case Study 3

The patient has COPD and is struggling with the activity limitations caused by the COPD. It is having negative effects on her family, work, and sleep.

Interaction Without Motivational Interviewing

Nurse: Good morning. How have you been?

Patient: Not so good. I have been having such a hard time breathing that it's difficult to do anything.

Nurse: That's a common problem for people with COPD.

Patient: So, what am I supposed to do?

Nurse: Well, let me look at what medications you are taking. How often do you feel you need something to help you breathe?

Patient: I only have about an hour after I take my medicine, and I need it again.

Nurse: I see. Well, it looks like you are on the maximum doses of everything you take. You might want to talk to the doctor about this. You might need different medication.

Patient: So, there is nothing else I can do?

Nurse: You should try to rest when you can and cluster your activities so you have plenty of time to rest.

Patient: Oh.

Motivational Interviewing Interaction

Nurse: Good morning. How have you been feeling?

Patient: Not so good. I feel so short of breath lately that I can't do much of anything.

Nurse: That must be frightening to feel that way.

Patient: Yes, it is. And I don't know what I can do.

Nurse: Could you share a little more about what's been going on?

Patient: It has been getting worse over the past few weeks. I get so tired and short of breath that it's not easy to work or do the housework. My husband is getting so tired of having to go for walks by himself. We used to always go together, but I just can't make it.

Nurse: The difficulty breathing is affecting every aspect of your life.

Patient: Yes, it is. I'm just so upset about it. I do everything I'm supposed to. I listen to what my doctor tells me. I just don't know what to do.

Nurse: You have worked very hard to manage your COPD. It's very disappointing to put in so much effort and see negative results.

Patient: I have. I really have tried so hard.

Nurse: It's like sewing a quilt by hand, square by square, and then it falls apart.

Patient: That is it. That is how it feels.

Nurse: You should be proud of all you have done to manage your COPD. I understand you still want it better. You want to be able to breathe easier.

Patient: I do, but there is nothing else I can do. (Ambivalence)

Nurse: Tell me how you managed episodes like this when you were first diagnosed.

Patient: Well, I guess I tried some stress management because I found that when I was stressed, it really did make my breathing worse. I had a lot to be stressed about back then.

Nurse: In this day and age it is not easy to be stress free.

Patient: You can say that again. There is always something I'm stressed about, whether it is my husband's health, my kids needing me, or worrying about my grandson Richard, who hasn't been well lately.

Nurse: Let's take a moment to recap. You have been having some increased shortness of breath. When you were first diagnosed, you found that stress reduction helped your symptoms. You recognize you have some stressors in your life right now. I'm curious what stress management might do for you now.

Patient: I don't know, but it certainly seems like it would help. I can't believe I didn't think of that. (Change talk)

Nurse: You had all the pieces there. I'm here to help you put together the puzzle.

Discussion

In the previous two scenarios the patient is struggling with being too short of breath to do her normal daily activities. In the first scenario although the nurse tried to assess the medication regimen, she may have considered asking the patient what was most difficult about dealing with the shortness of breath. The patient was not able to fully express what challenges she was facing. When the problem is not revealed, the patient does not get the opportunity to objectively evaluate the situation and find solutions to the perceived problems. The nurse must not assume what behaviors need to be changed, tell the patient what he or she must do, or leave the patient feeling hopeless. This patient left the first scenario feeling as if the situation was out of her control. This leads to acceptance of the problem and belief that there is nothing she can change to improve the situation.

In the second scenario the nurse used motivational interviewing to help the patient evaluate her situation and what has helped her overcome her current obstacle in the past. When the patients can look back and make a connection with a positive behavior and positive result, they can then compare with their current situation to see if it could be a potential solution. Drawing on past positive experiences can provide the necessary motivation the patient needs to accomplish a goal. In this case the goal was for the patient to have something she could do to help manage her symptoms. Unfortunately, COPD is chronic and the symptoms can worsen over time; medication management may not always be sufficient. Helping patients find another technique they can perform independently increases their self-efficacy. The nurse used a metaphor to relate the patient's problem. This provided reassurance that the nurse understood what the patient was experiencing. Metaphors are not as easy to incorporate into the conversation as some other motivational interviewing tactics. Figure 13-1 provides examples of metaphors. The use of motivational interviewing tactics allowed this patient to get to the source of the problem and discuss some options she had to improve the situation.

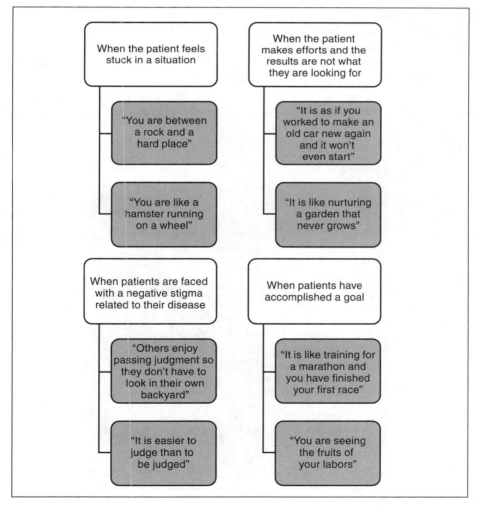

Figure 13-1 Metaphors

PRACTICE TOOLS (FIGURE 13-2)

1. Have the patient envision a positive example. Creating a picture in the mind of a positive situation can help provide insight into ideas to overcome barriers to treatment. Simple, small steps can be elucidated and a new perspective can be found. Patients may get so caught up in the negative side of things they do not take the time to look for the positive. When they find the positive, they can then build on it to make a stronger foundation from which to manage their disease.
2. It is important to support self-efficacy to build self-confidence. When we don't have faith in ourselves, we are less likely to take action. Sometimes a simple word of praise can boost the patient's feelings of self-efficacy. A vote of confidence from the nurse can be the one piece of conversation patients take with them when they leave the encounter. The patient should leave each encounter feeling validated.

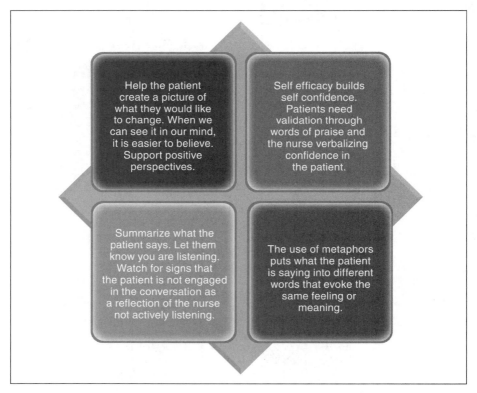

Figure 13-2   Practice Tools

3. Summarizing information the patient shares with you reinforces that you are really listening to what they have to say. If the patient doesn't feel heard, he or she will stop sharing. It is important to keep the conversation flowing. When a patient becomes quiet and backs away from the conversation, the nurse has demonstrated a lack of interest, understanding, or support of the patient.

4. Use metaphors. Motivational interviewing tactics are designed to help the patient feel validation and empathy. The use of metaphors is one of these tactics. It is a way of showing the patient that we understand his or her perspective. We can put it into other words that evoke the same feeling or meaning. This tactic can be more challenging because it is not always easy to come up with a metaphor for every situation.

5. Use available resources:
   - American Lung Association
   - Centers for Disease Control and Prevention
   - Cystic Fibrosis Foundation
   - Environmental Protection Agency: Asthma
   - National Asthma Control Program
   - National Asthma Education and Prevention Program
   - National Center for Environmental Health
   - National Heart, Lung, and Blood Institute
   - National Institute of Allergy and Infectious Diseases
   - Society for Public Health Education
   - World Health Organization

TAKE-AWAY POINTS

1. Pulmonary disorders contribute to many deaths, healthcare dollars spent, and missed days at school and work. The significance of the impact on our nation's health is unimaginable. Healthy People 2010 focuses on this group of disorders because of the effect it has on our health. This initiative prompted the development of various programs to help accomplish these goals.

2. Nonadherence to medications is very common in patients with a chronic pulmonary disorder. Various reasons for this were covered earlier in this chapter. A nonjudgmental approach is necessary to support patients as they evaluate their personal situation and explore their barriers and obstacles.

3. It is important to recognize that patients have the answers within themselves. They bring the information to the table and the nurse is present to help them sort it out and find a system that works for them. They are the experts of their life. The nurse does not know what their life is like until

he or she asks or encourages this discussion. Trust in your patients that they can find their own path.

4. The nurse's role is to help patients recognize triggers for exacerbation of their symptoms. Once identified, the patient can evaluate what he or she feels is reasonable to change, if anything, and then proceed to explore options for making changes. If we do not fully understand what is causing the problem, we cannot expect to find a solution.

SUMMARY

Motivational interviewing can be an effective tool in preventing and managing pulmonary disorders. Negative behaviors that contribute to exacerbations of chronic illness or acquiring acute illness should be identified. The nurse can help the patient explore what negative behaviors may be causing or contributing to the challenges the patient may be facing. In efforts to improve pulmonary health in the United States we must use effective tools within our nurse–patient interactions. If the patient chooses to change even one negative behavior to a positive behavior, it will increase the quality of life for that patient. Instead of making the patient revolve his or her life around the disorder, help the patient to manage the disorder around his or her life. Make the disease fit into the patient's lifestyle.

REFERENCES

Bartholomew, L., Parcel, G., Swank, P., & Czyzewski, D. (1993). Measuring self-efficacy expectations for the self-management of cystic fibrosis. *Chest, 103*(5), 1524–1530.

Elder, M. A., & Mellon, M. (2008). Long-term inhaled corticosteroid therapy in children and adolescents with persistent asthma: Facilitating adherence to guidelines-based therapy. *American Journal for Nurse Practitioners, 12*(11/12), 9–12, 16–18.

Elliott, R. (2006). Poor adherence to anti-inflammatory medication in asthma: Reasons, challenges, and strategies for improved disease management. *Disease Management Health Outcomes, 14*(4), 223–233.

Rubak, S., Sandboek, A., Lauritzen, T., & Christensen, B. (2005). Motivational interviewing: A systematic review and meta-analysis. *British Journal of General Practice, 55*(513), 303–312.

Wingrove, B. (2009). Pediatric respiratory infections. *Clinician Reviews, 19*(2), 20–26.

CHAPTER 14

Motivational Interviewing in Preventive Care

INTRODUCTION

We are currently in an age of **health maintenance**, **health promotion**, and **disease prevention**. The United States continues to have higher occurrences of chronic illness and preventable disease than is necessary, despite significant technology and resources. Healthy People 2010 was established in 1980 as a national initiative to promote healthy behaviors. Each decade a group of health experts get together and review data on our healthcare system and create goals to help improve the health of our nation. Currently, the Healthy People 2010 initiative is busy evaluating the outcomes of current goals, and there is work being done for Healthy People 2020. At the time of this writing goals and objectives are not available for Healthy People 2020. This information is planned to be available in late 2009 and early 2010.

As we prepare for a new set of goals and objectives, it is important to see how far we have come in attaining the goals of Healthy People 2010 in the areas of preventive care. We also look at recommendations from the **American Academy of Pediatrics (AAP)** and the **American Academy of Family Physicians (AAFP)** for preventive care. The focus on prevention is strong, and as nurses our role is to carry out these goals to promote a healthier nation.

Counseling patients about healthy behaviors is one objective under the Healthy People 2010 focus area of "Access to Quality Health Services." Data were obtained throughout the decade to evaluate performance of this goal. The statistical information from this source was retrieved on July 22, 2009 from the DATA2010-May 2009 edition (see http://wonder.cdc.gov/scripts/broker.exe).

Health behaviors that required counseling include (see http://wonder.cdc.gov/scripts/broker.exe)

- Physical activity (age 18 and older)
- Diet and nutrition (age 18 and older)
- Smoking cessation (age 18 and older)
- Risky drinking (age 18 and older)
- Unintended pregnancy (females aged 15–44)
- Prevention of sexually transmitted diseases (males and females aged 15–44)
- Management of menopause (women aged 45–57)

Ongoing wellness care is important to detect areas that require prevention measures or health maintenance. This level is important at all ages. Healthy People 2010 set forth goals to achieve routine care. Ninety-six percent of our population should be receiving routine health maintenance. As of 2006 we were falling short by 10%. When broken down to the pediatric population (age 17 and under) and the adult population (age 18 and over), we are clearly closer to our goal within the pediatric population. Ninety-four percent of children versus 83% of adults are receiving routine care. Part of this objective is also to achieve 85% of our population with a usual primary care provider. As of 2006, 78% of our population had achieved this goal (see http://wonder.cdc.gov/scripts/broker.exe).

Another task set forth to meet this goal is to achieve 7% of our population who have difficulties or delays in obtaining needed health care. In 2006 we had achieved 20%, which has actually increased from the baseline data of 12% in 1996. Emergency care is another area that can be delayed and result in physical harm. Healthy People 2010 is striving for only 1.5% of our adult population to struggle with these delays. By 2001 we had achieved this goal. There may be many reasons for delays, such as a decline in the number of healthcare providers available, lack of sufficient insurance to cover healthcare costs, or simply a lack of patient education about how and when to access health care (see http://wonder.cdc.gov/scripts/broker.exe).

Many conditions are preventable. Two areas of focus have been hospitalizations for uncontrolled diabetes and immunization-preventable pneumonia or influenza. With proper self-management of diabetes, many of these hospitalizations can be prevented. Through immunization, we could also prevent most cases of pneumonia and influenza. As of 2006 there were 8.4 admissions for uncontrolled diabetes per 10,000 population aged 18 to 64, with a target goal of 5.4 per 10,000 population. At the same time there were 7.6 hospitalizations for pneumonia or influenza per 10,000 population aged 65 and older, with a target goal of 7.9 per 10,000 population. This does not even include the numerous hospitalizations for younger populations (see http://wonder.cdc.gov/scripts/broker.exe).

Cancer prevention is an important area because of the impact it has on the health of our nation. Areas of counseling that are designated as part of achieving this goal include

- Smoking cessation
- Blood stool tests
- Proctoscopic examinations
- Mammograms
- Pap tests
- Physical activity

Not only is the counseling aspect important, but having these tests performed is even more important. Ninety-three percent of females aged 18 and older have ever received a Pap test. The goal is to reach 97% of this population. A target goal of 90% of this population having received a Pap test within the past 3 years was established. As of 2005 only 78% of the population could claim to have achieved this goal. We have a target goal of 33% of the population of those aged 50 and older to have had fecal occult blood testing that has not been met. A total of 17% of this population achieved this goal by 2005, the most recent data. A sigmoidoscopy is another way to screen for colorectal cancer. The target goal of 50% of the population aged 50 and older was met by 2005. For women age 40 and older, mammograms are important to increase early detection of breast cancer. The target goal for this population is 70%, and as of 2005 we achieved a 67% statistic (see http://wonder.cdc.gov/scripts/broker.exe).

Diabetes management is one of many areas proven to improve with proper education and evaluation. Healthy People 2010 set forth some specific objectives to be met in regards to diabetes. For those with diabetes, aged 18 and older, 60% should be receiving diabetes education. As of 1999, the most recent data available,

55% of this population was receiving such education. Medicare beneficiaries should be receiving annual microalbumin measurement to evaluate kidney function. A target goal was set at 14%. By 2006 we had surpassed the goal with 29% of this population having this evaluation done. To evaluate diabetes management, an A_{IC} test (now replaced with the **estimated average glucose**) is recommended twice a year. The goal is for those aged 18 and over, and in 2006, 64% of this population had achieved this. The target goal is 72%. Annual dilated eye exams are also recommended. The goal is for 76% of this same population to have this exam. In 2003, 58% of this population was having this test done biannually. The target goal for annual foot exams is set at 91%. By 2006 we had achieved only 68%. Prevention of heart disease through use of daily aspirin therapy is recommended for the diabetes population. A target of 30% of this population was set with our most current data showing only 20%, which was baseline data between 1999 and 2002 (see http://wonder.cdc.gov/scripts/broker.exe).

Our children spend a large portion of their time in school, and this is a place where they can consistently receive health education. Healthy People 2010 set forth many goals to be achieved in the school system. The following areas of education are recommended:

- Unintentional injury
- Violence
- Suicide
- Tobacco use and addiction
- Alcohol and other drug use
- Unintended pregnancy, HIV/AIDS, and sexually transmitted infections
- Unhealthy dietary patterns
- Inadequate physical activity
- Environmental health

Health risk behavior for college students is yet another area for education (see http://wonder.cdc.gov/scripts/broker.exe).

Our worksites are another area where we can achieve health promotion. Healthy People 2010 encourages a target of 75% of worksite health promotion programs. Our communities should also be offering health promotion programs. A target of 90% of adults 65 and older participating in this program has yet to be achieved. In 1998 the baseline data was set at 12%, and no further data were recorded at the time of this writing (see http://wonder.cdc.gov/scripts/broker.exe).

Unintended pregnancies and sexually transmitted diseases (STDs) weigh heavily on the U.S. healthcare system. Healthy People 2010 recognizes the importance of prevention in this area. The following areas have become a focus for improving these statistics:

- Contraceptive use
- Emergency contraception

- Male involvement in pregnancy prevention
- Pregnancy and STD prevention through condom use
- Pregnancy and STD prevention through condom and hormonal methods
- Prevention education: abstinence
- Prevention education: birth control methods
- HIV/AIDS prevention
- STD prevention

A goal of 90% insurance coverage for contraceptive supplies and services has been established. In 2002 baseline data of 86% was documented, with no further data available at the time of this writing (see http://wonder.cdc.gov/scripts/broker.exe).

Patient satisfaction with the healthcare services they receive is another important factor that can contribute to patients seeking preventive health care. Healthy People 2010 determined several areas of reported patient satisfaction in relation to their interactions with healthcare providers:

- Provider listens carefully to the patient
- Provider explains things so patients understand
- Provider shows respect for what the patient has to say
- Provider spends enough time with the patient

Little, if any, change has been noted since baseline data were obtained (see http://wonder.cdc.gov/scripts/broker.exe).

Healthy People 2010 set forth a goal of 90–95% immunization rate. Immunizations received should be in accordance with the recommended vaccine schedule set by the Committee on Infectious Diseases. Most recent data demonstrate a range of 68–93% of children and adolescents are receiving the recommended immunizations. Adults with high risk are only at an 18–66% rate of receiving immunizations. Vaccination is one of the simplest forms of prevention, and we should be reaching more of our population (see http://wonder.cdc.gov/ scripts/broker.exe).

Safety and injury is another focus area for Healthy People 2010. We have almost achieved the goal of decreasing injury-related emergency room visits to 108 per 1,000 standard population. The use of safety belts was at a rate of 82% in 2005, with a target goal of 92%. The use of child restraints in children 4 years of age and younger should be accomplished 100% of the time. In 2006 this was occurring 92% of the time. Motorcycle helmet use is at a 48% rate of occurrence. The goal for children using a bicycle helmet is 76% of this population. In 1998, 69% of children were wearing bicycle helmets. No further data were available in this report. Adult use of bicycle helmets was at a rate of 38% with a target goal of 42% (see http://wonder.cdc.gov/scripts/broker.exe).

Prevention of complications to mother or fetus during pregnancy is another way that we can improve health in the United States. Healthy People 2010 set forth goals of pregnant women abstaining from alcohol, binge drinking, cigarette smoking, and illicit drug use. Target goals range from 95% to 100%. Most recent data suggest success rates of 88–96% (see http://wonder.cdc.gov/scripts/broker.exe).

Maintaining a healthy weight can prevent health problems and improve current chronic health issues. A goal of 60% of adults aged 20 and older is to be at a healthy weight. Data from 2003–2006 demonstrated a rate of 32% falling within healthy weight guidelines. The target rate for obesity in this population is set for 15%, but we are at a 33% rate from the same set of data. The target goal for overweight and obesity in children is 5%. The data set from 2003 to 2006 revealed a rate of 17–18%. Many programs are available that focus on obesity and the need for healthy weight. Diet and nutrition are often an important aspect of managing medical conditions. Counseling on nutrition should be included in physician office visits. Healthy People 2010 strives for 75% of adults receiving such counseling. As of 2005, 35% of patients in this population received nutrition counseling (see http://wonder.cdc.gov/scripts/broker.exe).

Physical activity is another component of health care that can prevent illness or complications of illness. The worksite is one place this can be encouraged. Healthy People 2010 set a target goal of 75% of worksites providing a physical activity program. Walking is encouraged for transportation. Twenty-five percent of adults and 50% of children should be walking on trips of 1 mile or less. Most current data state we are approximately half way to the target goals. Bicycling for trips 5 miles or less should be used by 2% of adults and 5% of children. The most current data have decreased from baseline data, leaving us further to go to reach the target (see http://wonder.cdc.gov/scripts/broker.exe).

Asthma is another chronic condition that can benefit from self-management. To achieve proper self-management skills, Healthy People 2010 encourages patient education, written asthma action plans, adequate instruction for use of inhalers, education on early signs, symptoms and responses to asthma episodes, and assistance in reduction of symptom triggers or environmental risk factors (see http://wonder.cdc.gov/scripts/broker.exe).

Smoking cessation programs have become more readily available due to the Healthy People 2010 goals. A target goal of 80% was developed for smoking cessation attempts made by adults. In 2006 and 2007 we had a rate of 47%. At that time we also had a rate of 57% for the adolescent population, with a target goal of 64%. Coverage for nicotine dependency is lacking. A target goal for coverage from managed care organizations was set at 100% and Medicaid program coverage at 51%. In 1997–1998 baseline data were established at 75% coverage by managed care organizations and 24% Medicaid program coverage. No further data were available in this report (see http://wonder.cdc.gov/scripts/broker.exe).

The AAP has combined efforts with **Bright Futures**, an initiative for prevention and health promotion in pediatrics, to produce guidelines for the frequency of visits and what tasks should be performed depending on the age. (See

Figure 14-1 for guidelines on wellness visits.) This can be accessed through the AAP website (www.aap.org). "Bright Futures is a set of principles, strategies, and tools that are theory based, evidence driven, and systems oriented that can be used to improve the health and well-being of all children through culturally appropriate interventions that address their current and emerging health promotion needs at the family, clinical practice, community, health system, and policy levels" (Hagan, Shaw, & Duncan, 2008). Areas covered in the recommendations are as follows:

- Initial and interval history (past medical history, family history and social history)

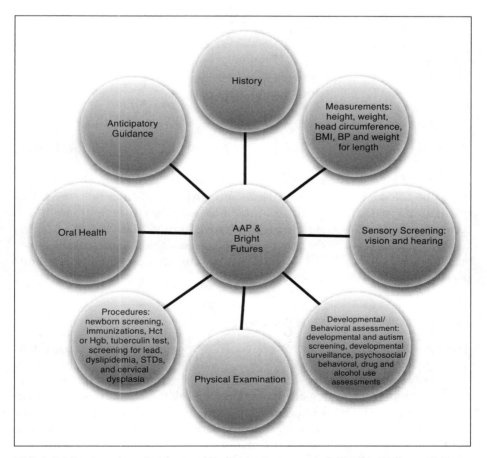

Figure 14-1   American Academy of Pediatrics Recommendation for Wellness Visits

Source: Adapted from American Academy of Pediatrics, 2008.

- Height and weight
- Head circumference (first 2 years)
- Weight for length
- Body mass index
- Blood pressure
- Vision and hearing screening
- Developmental screening and surveillance
- Autism screening
- Psychosocial/behavioral assessment
- Alcohol and drug use assessment
- Physical examination
- Newborn screening
- Immunizations
- Hemoglobin or hematocrit
- Lead screening
- Tuberculosis screening
- Screening for dyslipidemia
- Screening for STDs and cervical dysplasia
- Oral health
- Anticipatory guidance

Not all these tasks are recommended for every visit (Hagan, Shaw, & Duncan, 2008).

The AAFP also has recommendations for preventive health. These recommendations are for patients of all ages. Within these guidelines there are markers that designate the level of recommendation: strongly recommend (SR), recommend (R), no recommendation (NR), recommend against (RA), have insufficient evidence (I), or the healthy behavior is desirable but effectiveness is not yet determined (I-HB) (Table 14-1). These recommendations help to guide our practice of preventive care (AAFP, 2009).

CHALLENGES IN PREVENTIVE CARE

There are many challenges in preventive care. Preventive care is most consistent in the pediatric population simply because immunizations are a part of many visits and required to attend school. Schools require routine physical examinations for children to participate in school. Although these requirements help to ensure preventive visits are maintained for this population, some children do not stay on schedule for recommended visits. There are many reasons for this, such as religious and personal beliefs that parents hold against immunizations, lack of insurance coverage, and parental negligence. As we look forward to health-

Table 14-1. American Academy of Family Physicians Preventive Care Measures That
Are Recommended (R) or Strongly Recommended (SR)

- One time screening for abdominal aortic aneurysm by ultrasound in men aged
  65–75 who have a history of smoking (R)
- Counseling all parents and children over 2 years of age about prevention of
  accidental injuries (R)
- Screening and behavioral counseling to reduce alcohol misuse in all adults,
  including pregnant women (R)
- Screening for asymptomatic bacteriuria by urine culture, for pregnant women
  between 12–16 weeks gestation or at first prenatal visit, if later than 16 weeks (SR)
- Behavioral counseling to prevent STDs in all sexually active adolescents and adults
  who are at risk for STDs (R)
- Women, 40 and older, to have a mammogram every 1–2 years to screen for breast
  cancer (R)
- Referral to genetic counseling for women who have a family history that reveals
  increased risk for breast cancer gene mutations (R)
- Promotion and support of breastfeeding (R)
- Pap smear at least every 3 years to screen for cervical cancer for women who have
  ever had sex and have a cervix (SR)
- Screening for chlamydia in all women 24 and younger who are sexually active and
  older, nonpregnant women who are at risk (SR)
- Screening for chlamydia in all pregnant women 24 and younger and older pregnant
  women who have increased risk (R)
- Screening for colorectal cancer through stool for hemoccult blood, sigmoidoscopy,
  or colonoscopy in adults aged 50–75 (SR)
- Screening for congenital hypothyroidism in newborns (SR)
- Screening for congenital rubella syndrome through history, serology, or
  immunization of women of childbearing age (R)
- The use of aspirin in men aged 45–79 when the benefit to reduce myocardial
  infarction outweighs the risk of gastrointestinal bleeding (SR)
- The use of aspirin in women aged 55–79 when the benefit to reduce myocardial
  infarction outweighs the risk of gastrointestinal bleeding (SR)
- Fluoride supplementation from 6 months to 16 years for those children who do not
  have fluoride in their water supply (SR)
- Depression screening for all adults (R)
- Screening for type 2 diabetes in adults with asymptomatic blood pressure higher
  than 135/80 mm Hg, with or without medication (R)
- Immunize all children against diphtheria, *H. influenza* type b, hepatitis A, hepatitis
  B, influenza, measles, mumps, rubella, meningococcal, pertussis, pneumococcal,
  poliomyelitis, tetanus, and varicella (SR)

continues

Table 14-1. American Academy of Family Physicians Preventive Care Measures That Are Recommended (R) or Strongly Recommended (SR)—*continued*

- Immunize adults against diphtheria, tetanus (SR), and varicella (R if no previous disease or vaccination)
- Immunize at risk adults against hepatitis A, hepatitis B, influenza, measles, mumps, rubella, meningococcal, and pneumococcal (R and SR)
- Immunize adults > 50 years against influenza and adults > 65 against pneumococcal (R)
- Prophylactic medication in neonates to protect against gonococcal ophthalmia neonatorum (SR)
- Screening of all sexually active women and pregnant women for gonorrhea if they are at increased risk (R)
- Behavioral dietary counseling for adults with hyperlipidemia and other cardiac risk factors and diet-related chronic disease (R)
- Screening elderly for hearing impairment (R)
- Screening for hearing loss in all newborn infants (R)
- Screening for hepatitis B virus in pregnant women at their first prenatal visit (SR)
- Screening for high blood pressure in adults 18 and older (SR)
- Screening for HIV in adolescents and adults at increased risk (SR)
- Screening for HIV in pregnant women (R)
- Screening for iron deficiency anemia in asymptomatic pregnant women (R)
- Screening men 35 and older for lipid disorders (SR)
- Screening women 20 and older and men 25–35 for lipid disorders if they are at increased risk (R and SR)
- Prescribing 0.4–0.8 mg of folic acid to women of childbearing age and at least 1 month before conception through the first trimester for those planning to become pregnant (R and SR)
- Prescribing 4 mg of folic acid to women planning to become pregnant with previous pregnancy resulting in a neural tube defect, to be taken at least 1–3 months before conception and throughout the first trimester (SR)
- Screening all adult patients for obesity; for those who are obese offer counseling and behavioral interventions to promote sustained weight loss (more than one session a month for at least 3 months) (R)
- Screening women 65 and older for osteoporosis, women 60 and older for increased risk for osteoporotic fractures, and counseling females 11 and older about maintaining adequate calcium intake to prevent osteoporosis (R)
- Referral to genetic counseling for any woman whose family history suggests increased risk of genetic mutations that contribute to ovarian cancer (R)
- Screening for phenylketonuria in newborns (SR)
- Rh (D) blood typing and antibody testing for all pregnant women at the first prenatal visit and repeated Rh (D) negative women at 24–28 weeks' gestation (SR and R)

Table 14-1. American Academy of Family Physicians Preventive Care Measures That Are Recommended (R) or Strongly Recommended (SR)—*continued*

- Counsel smoking parents about the harmful effects of smoking and children's health (SR)
- Screening for sickle cell in all newborns (SR)
- Screening all pregnant women and those at increased risk for syphilis (SR)
- Screening for abnormal thyroid function in the neonate (SR)
- Screening all adults, including pregnant women, for tobacco use and provide smoking cessation interventions (SR)
- Screening for tuberculosis through the use of the Mantoux test for those at risk (SR)
- Vision screening in all children less than 5 and in elderly adults (R)

Source: From American Academy of Family Physicians (2009).

care reform and depend on our current ability to keep children covered by state health insurance programs, this should improve.

The adolescent population also does well in maintaining most preventive care. Schools continue to require routine physical exams and updated immunizations. Areas that are lacking yet also improving are risky behaviors of smoking, illicit drug use, and sexual behaviors that can lead to pregnancy and/or STDs. Schools have taken a role in educating adolescents in these areas. During preventive care visits healthcare providers also discuss these issues as part of anticipatory guidance. Parents and adolescents must also take an active role in preventing acute and chronic issues. National campaigns are advertised on television directed at parents and adolescents in hopes to prevent risky behaviors.

It is more challenging to reach the young adult population for preventive care. This population tends to be healthy and does not have routine health care. They seek out health care for minor illnesses, pregnancy or contraception, injuries, or physical exams for employment. It is crucial to reach this population to help prevent future health problems. The choices being made during this time will impact their future health. "Many of the choices young adults make, if not positive ones, will be difficult to modify later" (Bastable, 2006, p. 127). Other priorities interfere with seeking routine preventive care. This population is busy establishing independence, beginning careers, and relationships. The focus is the here and now, not their future health.

As adults age they become more focused on their health, especially when they develop a chronic health issue. Many physical changes occur during this stage of life. Maintaining health tends to be a greater focus than prevention, but prevention becomes a part of health maintenance. This population goes through many changes in regards to raising families and taking care of elderly parents.

Often, their careers are well established and retirement is before them. There are a lot of emotional adjustments to the changes an adult faces. Stress can significantly impact their overall health if they have not yet learned to cope with stress in a positive manner. Many adults provide care to family members who may have a chronic illness. They find it difficult to focus on their own health because they are busy caring for others. Health care is often sought when there are symptoms that can no longer be prevented.

Insurance coverage, access to health care, and trust in healthcare providers all interfere with preventive care. Until we have better insurance coverage or access to health insurance that is affordable, we will continue to face challenges in providing adequate preventive care. Establishing a trusting relationship with a healthcare provider is also important to ensure routine preventive healthcare visits. This is one reason it is important to take the time to establish a rapport with the patient. If they feel comfortable and safe and can trust in what you say, they are more likely to return.

BENEFITS TO MODIFYING BEHAVIOR TO PREVENT ILLNESS AND INJURY

It has been well established that smoking, lack of exercise, poor nutrition, and misuse of alcohol are modifiable risk factors for a variety of chronic diseases and mortality in the United States (Aspy et al., 2008; Bodenheimer & Handley, 2009; Flocke, Kelly, & Highland, 2009; Holtrop et al., in press). Prevention of these and other modifiable behaviors can improve health in the United States by reducing these risk factors. Nutrition counseling, smoking cessation, increasing physical activity, and reducing the overuse and dependence on alcohol should be topics of conversation at every primary care visit. There is no debate that counseling and behavior modification are beneficial. What is debatable is the ability to accomplish this in all healthcare settings. The fast pace of an emergency room, over-scheduling in primary care, and increased workload for nurses interfere with consistent preventive care services. Motivational interviewing offers a skill set to accomplish behavior change in various settings in which there is little time to work. Brief interventions can be accommodated by motivational interviewing techniques and result in positive behavior change.

In one study motivational interviewing was used to enhance weight loss through change in behavior (DiMarco, Klein, Clark, & Wilson, 2009). Overweight patients were provided half-hour to 1-hour blocks of time to interact with the therapist on eight separate occasions. Those who were part of the motivational interviewing group demonstrated superiority in areas of control over eating and eating concern, such as guilt over eating and fear of losing control over eating. Improving patient's eating patterns and behaviors can greatly improve the rate of obesity and decrease the risk of diabetes, cardiovascular disease, and sleep and joint disorders. There was less of a dropout rate in the group who participated in motivational interviewing, which increases the success of improving healthy eating behaviors (DiMarco et al., 2009).

Physical activity is another modifiable behavior that can have a positive impact on an individual's health. Studies have also shown motivational interviewing to be effective in promoting behavior change that leads to increased physical activity. One study looked at long-term cancer survivors and how motivational interviewing impacted behavior change to increase physical activity. The authors also looked at self-efficacy and how that impacts the success rate of improving health behaviors. "The synergy between self-efficacy and motivational interviewing counseling has been proposed as the main mechanism by which behavior change occurs, and the findings of this study provide evidence that is true in increasing physical activity in cancer survivors and, perhaps, in all persons" (Bennett, Lyons, Winters-Stone, Nail, & Scherer, 2007, p. 26).

In another study about methods to improve physical activity, lifestyle intervention was compared with structured group activity in older adults. It was found that lifestyle intervention was more effective in promoting and sustaining increased physical activity (Opdenacker, Boen, Coorevits, & Delecluse, 2008). Increased physical activity in this population decreases immobility, decreases complications of chronic illness, and increases general health, in addition to improving quality of life.

The importance of smoking cessation is widely known. The media tells us all the negative effects of tobacco use. Many programs promote smoking cessation, through community programs, statewide initiatives, and nationwide programs. You can access information through the Internet, by written material, and from your physician. Quitting smoking has tremendous health benefits and can prevent a variety of chronic diseases, such as lung diseases and cardiovascular diseases. "Smoking cessation is also predicted to increase population-wide life expectancy by 1 year and the life expectancy of the individual smoker by several years" (Cole, 2001, p. 156).

CASE STUDIES

The following case studies show how motivational interviewing can be used in conversations about preventive care in contrast with non-motivational interviewing techniques.

Case Study 1

The patient has diabetes and is here for a routine visit. He struggles with getting exercise, and it is affecting his blood glucose levels, increasing his risk for long-term complications.

Interaction Without Motivational Interviewing

Nurse: Good morning. How are you?

Patient: I'm doing well.

Nurse: At the last visit I see we were talking about exercise and how important it is to help keep your blood sugars stable.

Patient: That's right.

Nurse: So, how is the exercise?

Patient: I try.

Nurse: How often are you exercising?

Patient: Oh, you know; a walk here and there.

Nurse: Getting routine exercise is very important, especially when you have diabetes. Your diabetes control is not where it needs to be. If you try exercising, you will see an improvement.

Patient: Okay.

Motivational Interviewing Interaction

Nurse: Good morning. How are you?

Patient: I'm doing well.

Nurse: I see that we were talking about exercise at the last visit. We can go back to that or we can talk about anything else you are concerned about.

Patient: Well, I can't see how exercise can help me. I tried to stay on a routine and I still don't have control over my blood sugars. (Resistance)

Nurse: You are frustrated.

Patient: Of course I'm frustrated. I worked hard and it didn't make a difference.

Nurse: You saw a benefit to exercising and you put a lot of effort into it. Tell me what you found positive in your experience.

Patient: Well, I felt better and had more energy.

Nurse: Your efforts paid off in how you felt. I'm curious about what you found negative about your experience with exercise.

Patient: The numbers were pretty good, but my A_{Ic} didn't improve much. I thought I would be doing better with the diabetes. (Ambivalence)

Nurse: Let me understand. You know the benefits of having exercise in your daily routine, you were feeling healthier, and your blood glucose readings were improving.

Patient: That's right. But then you tell me my A_{Ic} and I'm not even close to where I need to be.

Nurse: Tell me about where you feel you need to be.

Patient: I need my A_{Ic} to be <7%. I'm still at 8.7%.

Nurse: Paint me a picture. Show me how you want to reach your goal and how long you think is realistic to attain your goal.

Patient: I have been eating very well and I want to have more of a routine for exercise. I know those two things will help my blood sugars. I want to be there right now. I want to have good control. But I guess it will take some time. What would you think is a reasonable amount of time to get where I want to be? (Change talk)

Nurse: Well, we know the A_{Ic} is a glucose average over a 2- to 3-month period of time. With consistent healthy nutrition and routine exercise, you could reasonably attain your goal over a 3-month period of time, or at least get close to your goal.

Patient: So, I could definitely reach my goal within 6 months.

Nurse: I am confident that once you get into a routine, you will be successful.

Discussion

In the previous two scenarios a patient with a chronic illness can greatly benefit from routine exercise. The patient is not getting as much exercise as he should to reap the benefits and improve his overall health. In the first scenario the nurse does not explore why the patient is not getting enough exercise. The nurse tells the patient to get routine exercise. This is too vague. A patient needs a better understanding of what routine exercise means. Telling a patient what to do without determining if it is possible results in resistance from the patient and he or she will not likely comply. The first scenario demonstrates ineffective communication that resulted in the patient becoming passive, and you can sense that nothing is going to change with this patient's activity level.

In the second scenario the nurse used motivational interviewing techniques. The patient was frustrated because he had expected more improvement for the amount of effort he put into an exercise routine. The nurse guided the patient as he explored positive and negative aspects of exercising. He was frustrated to see less than desirable results from his efforts. By exploring the positive aspects of exercising, the patient was able to recognize that he had felt better physically. It is important to help patients focus on the positive aspects because it is often the negatives that drive us and prevent behavior change.

Case Study 2

The patient is a child who is new to the pediatric practice. He is here for a routine exam and immunizations.

Interaction Without Motivational Interviewing

> Nurse: Good morning. How has Cobie been doing?
>
> Parent: Oh, he's good. We haven't had any problems.
>
> Nurse: Today we are doing his physical. Do you have any concerns?
>
> Parent: Not really.
>
> Nurse: At the end of the physical, I will give him his immunizations.
>
> Parent: Oh, I don't want him to have his immunizations.
>
> Nurse: Why not?
>
> Parent: Too many bad things can happen from those vaccines.
>
> Nurse: More benefits come from vaccines than side effects. He really needs to have them.
>
> Parent: No. I don't want him to have them.
>
> Nurse: Your child needs the immunizations and is at greater risk if he doesn't have them.
>
> Parent: I don't want him to have the immunizations and that is it.

Motivational Interviewing Interaction

> Nurse: Good morning. How has Cobie been?
>
> Parent: He has been good. He hasn't had any problems.
>
> Nurse: Today we are doing his physical. Do you have any concerns?
>
> Parent: Not really.
>
> Nurse: After we do the physical exam, we can do the immunizations.
>
> Parent: I would rather not do the immunizations.
>
> Nurse: Share with me the concerns you are having.
>
> Parent: Well, I have heard too much about the bad things that can happen.
>
> Nurse: Tell me about that.
>
> Parent: I've heard that some of these vaccines can cause autism and I don't want to take that chance. One of my friends has a child with autism, and it has to be from the vaccines. No one else in their family has ever had it.
>
> Nurse: You understand autism to be genetic or caused by vaccines.
>
> Parent: Yes, I do.
>
> Nurse: Would you like me to share with you a little more information about autism and vaccines?
>
> Parent: Sure, but I don't know if it will change my mind.
>
> Nurse: Well, we know from many studies that there is no definite link between vaccines and autism. What happens is that autism symptoms can develop around the same time as certain vaccines are administered. Often,

there are symptoms before this time, but they are subtle. Cobie shows no sign of autism at this point.

Parent: I do feel like he is right where he is supposed to be. But I can't help but be concerned.

Nurse: Well, let's look at the flip side of things. What do you think might happen if he doesn't have the vaccine?

Parent: I guess there is a chance he could end up with the disease you are trying to protect him against.

Nurse: On one hand, you feel he could become autistic if he gets the immunizations, but on the other hand, you want to protect him from other serious diseases.

Parent: That's all I want to do is to protect him.

Nurse: It is a tough decision that all of us, as parents, must make. We all struggle with making the right choices for our children. We don't want our children to develop autism, measles, mumps or rubella, or any of the other diseases we now have vaccines for.

Parent: So, you understand my concerns?

Nurse: Yes, I do. Being a parent means we have to really weigh the risks and the benefits of what we choose for our children. It's been a long road, but we have come to a point where we rarely see outbreaks of vaccine-preventable diseases. People who support the autism debate are well publicized, and we tend to be swayed by what we see on television or hear in the news.

Parent: That is true. And I would hate for my son to develop a deadly disease that I could have prevented by having him immunized.

Nurse: We have talked about the pros and cons to immunizing. I am curious if you have any other concerns about the vaccines.

Parent: No. I think you covered it all. I appreciate you taking the time and understanding my concerns.

Nurse: Being a parent means making difficult decisions and for you it happens to be about the vaccines. I hope I clarified enough so you can make a decision about what you feel is best for Cobie.

Parent: I think so. I will go ahead and have him get the vaccines and we'll see how it goes.

Nurse: Okay. How about we proceed with the exam?

Discussion

In the previous two scenarios the parent does not want her son to receive immunizations. In the first scenario the nurse argues that the child needs the immunizations, and it is better to risk the potential side effects than to suffer the possible consequences of not being immunized. The parent was defensive and not interested in discussion about the immunizations. The nurse did not promote therapeutic communication. Instead, she triggered the parent's defensive stance and did not take cues from the parent when she became resistant.

In the second scenario the nurse hears the parent has concerns and further assessed those concerns. With permission, she shared additional information so the parent could make an informed decision. Together they looked at the pros and cons of immunizing the child. The parent was appreciative of the nurse's empathy and open discussion about her concerns. There was a more positive tone to the conversation because the nurse was not simply telling the parent about the importance of immunizing but exploring the issue together. The nurse did not act superior and let the parent know that she, too, has difficulty making choices for her children and that this is a normal phenomenon. The parent was not alone in the process of exploring the core of the issue. The nurse walked beside the parent and the parent was then able to make the decision. There may be times the parent continues to refuse vaccines despite a conversation such as this. Within the motivational interviewing framework, the nurse must accept the parent's choices but at the same time ensure the parent has appropriate information to make an informed decision.

Case Study 3

The patient is here for a prenatal visit. She is struggling with quitting smoking. The nurse recognizes the potential risks to the mother and the child.

Interaction Without Motivational Interviewing

Nurse: Good morning. How are you doing?

Patient: I'm pretty good.

Nurse: Do you mind if I take a moment to go over your last visit with you?

Patient: That is fine.

Nurse: I see you are taking the prenatal vitamins. You haven't had any significant problems during the pregnancy up to this point. And at the last visit, you were still smoking. How has that been going for you?

Patient: Well, I have cut down, but it's hard to stop completely.

Nurse: I'm sure you have heard the statistics before and know that every cigarette puts you and the baby at risk for complications.

Patient: (silent)

Nurse: It is not too late to quit. I see the doctor discussed this with you at the last visit. We really need to work on this so you can prevent a premature birth and unhealthy baby.

Patient: I know. (starts to cry)

Nurse: There must be things you can do to distract yourself so you don't smoke.

Patient: I have tried different things and they just don't work. I just can't help it.

Nurse: You have a choice. Quitting smoking now is the best thing you can do for you and your baby.

Patient: I know.

Nurse: We have you coming back in about a month. I want you to work on it and we will talk again at the next visit.

Patient: Okay.

Motivational Interviewing Interaction

Nurse: Good morning. How are you doing?

Patient: I'm pretty good.

Nurse: Do you mind if I take a moment to go over your last visit with you?

Patient: That is fine.

Nurse: I see you are taking the prenatal vitamins. You haven't had any significant problems during the pregnancy up to this point. And at the last visit, you were still smoking. How has that been going for you?

Patient: Well, I have cut down, but it's hard to stop completely. (Resistance)

Nurse: There is always something that prevents us from stopping a bad habit. It is usually something we see as positive about it, despite the negatives.

Patient: There are some days that I can do really well because every time I want a cigarette, I think about the baby and I don't have one. But I've been under a lot of stress and it's hard not to pick up a cigarette when I'm stressed out. (Ambivalence)

Nurse: You find smoking helps to decrease the stress.

Patient: Not exactly. It just helps to calm my nerves.

Nurse: I'm wondering what you think might happen if you don't have a cigarette when you are feeling that stressed.

Patient: I get very irritable and I'm afraid I'm going to drive my husband away. He is under enough stress because he just lost his job and when I get irritable, we end up fighting. Then I get even more stressed out because we are fighting.

Nurse: You are afraid that if you don't have the cigarettes to help calm you that you and your husband will argue. You are concerned about the effect it might have on your marriage.

Patient: That is true. I just wish I didn't get irritable and feel like I need a cigarette.

Nurse: Everyone has different ways of managing stress. What are your thoughts about other things you can do when you feel stressed?

Patient: I don't know. I have thought about taking a yoga class because I've heard that is good to help with stress. I used to go running, but I can't exactly run right now.

Nurse: So, some form of exercise or physical activity helps you to feel calm.

Patient: Yes, I guess it has in the past.

Nurse: (silent)

Patient: I've always enjoyed walking, running, swimming, and such. I could try some of these things like walking and swimming. There shouldn't be any problem doing those things while I'm pregnant. (Change talk)

Nurse: No. It is actually good to exercise while you are pregnant. Many people find they feel better with exercise. On a scale of 1 to 10, how ready are you to try an exercise plan to help you quit smoking?

Patient: I would say about an 8 or 9.

Nurse: What might be your first steps?

Patient: I'm thinking I should try to plan at least two walks a day, or get in the pool for a little while each day. And when I am feeling stressed out, maybe I can go walk the dog. My husband I can do that together and maybe it will help us both to deal with stress.

Nurse: That sounds like a great idea. Having an idea of what to do when the urge to smoke is there, will help you to be successful. I am confident that you can quit.

Patient: Thank you. I really am going to try this out.

Discussion

The previous two scenarios look at the difficult topic of smoking cessation. This particular case is even more difficult because the patient is pregnant. The many risks of smoking during pregnancy can drive the nurse to be more direct about what they believe needs to be done. Our personal beliefs can interfere with maintaining an objective perspective and allowing the patient to make that choice. In the first scenario the nurse pushes the importance of quitting by telling the patient about the negative effects of smoking during pregnancy. The nurse does not explore why it is so challenging for this particular patient to quit smoking. The patient kept saying "I know," and this reinforces the claim that our patients often know what needs to be done, but they struggle with the how and the motivation to follow through. The patient became passive in this scenario and was not able to commit to any plan to quit smoking, clearly making it an ineffective communication.

In the second scenario the nurse helps the patient to explore the challenges in quitting smoking and ways to avoid smoking. For this patient it is exercise that is helpful. The nurse used motivational interviewing skills and was able to discover some of the deeper challenges the patient is facing in regard to what is contributing to the stress that she feels drives her to smoke. The patient was able to come up with a plan that could improve the situation with her husband by including him when she gets physical activity. The Likert scale was used in this interaction. The patient reported a high level of motivation, so the nurse did not further explore why she was not more or less motivated. The patient already had motivation, so the next step was guiding the patient to develop a plan. The nurse remained nonjudgmental and was successful in helping the patient to move toward healthy behavior change.

PRACTICE TOOLS (FIGURE 14-2)

1. For every behavior there are positive and negative results. It is important to help the patient closely evaluate how he or she feels when performing a specific behavior. Find out what feels good about the behavior and explore what the downside is to having the behavior. Further exploring what is positive and negative about making the behavior change can reveal a lot about a person. Find out what is meaningful to the patient. Just as we do not want our patients to make uninformed decisions, we should not assume we know what the patient desires. We must inform ourselves about the patient through the use of motivational interviewing techniques.

2. It is okay to let the patient know that you have similar challenges. The patient has respect for the nurse that shares an understanding of how difficult some choices are to make. The nurse should not share too much personal information because the conversation then becomes about the nurse. The interaction must remain patient centered. When the nurse reveals vulnerability in personal decision making, the patient can develop respect for the nurse and see the nurse as human and not as superior. It is important to walk the path with the patient and not be the one leading the way.

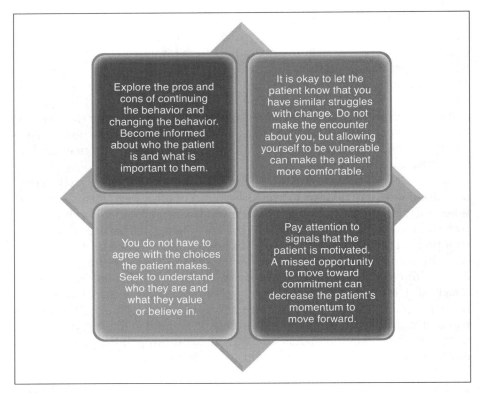

Figure 14-2 Practice Tools

3. Recognize that nurses cannot always agree with the choices a patient makes. A patient's choice may go against everything in which we personally believe. Showing judgment closes the door to any future opportunities to promote behavior change with that patient. Our job is not to close doors but to open them. Maintaining a conversational tone is more successful for establishing a rapport with the patient than informing the patient about what needs to be different to improve his or her health. It is important to explore the patient's beliefs. Our goal is not to change a patient's religious or cultural beliefs but seek to understand them.

4. Pay attention to signals that the patient is motivated. Guiding the patient who is motivated toward making a plan can best be done when they show a high motivation level. We could easily explore the high level of motivation, but we would be passing up an opportunity to help the patient get

one step closer to making a change. When in doubt, reflect motivation to change back to the patient. The patient will let you know if you are wrong in your interpretation or not. It is okay to be wrong and may even be beneficial to attaining even more information that will provide insight into who this person is and what is important to him or her. This can guide the patient to that "ah-ha!" moment when they see and feel why it is important for change in behavior and feel an inner desire to make that change. The moment of clarity is when everything is aligned and it only seems right to move forward.

5. Use available resources:
   - American Academy of Family Physicians
   - American Academy of Pediatrics
   - American Association for Health Education
   - American College of Preventive Medicine
   - American Council on Exercise
   - American Public Health Association
   - American School Health Association
   - Association for Prevention Teaching and Research
   - Bright Futures
   - Coalition for Healthier Cities and Communities
   - Healthy People 2010, Healthy People 2020
   - National Alliance for Nutrition and Activity
   - National Association for Public Health Statistics and Information Systems
   - National Association for Public Worksite Health Promotion
   - National Association of State Boards of Education
   - National Center for Health Education
   - National Center for Tobacco-Free Kids
   - National Commission Against Drunk Driving
   - National Council on Patient Information and Education
   - National Environmental Health Association
   - National Healthy Mothers, Healthy Babies Coalition
   - National Newborn Screening and Genetics Resource Center
   - National Safety Council
   - Partnership for Prevention
   - Planned Parenthood Federation of America, Inc.
   - Public Health Institute
   - SAFE KIDS USA
   - Shape Up America!
   - Society for Public Health Education
   - U.S. Preventive Services Task Force

TAKE-AWAY POINTS

1. Preventive care is a concept that was deemed important long ago. We know that there are many ways to prevent injury and disease. We also know that the way to prevention is through behavior change. Behavior change is challenging to even the strongest people. To promote behavior change, we must create an environment that allows for open communication.
2. Motivational interviewing is an effective way to promote behavior change. Every healthy behavior decreases the risk of chronic illness and accidental injuries. Healthy People 2010 placed an emphasis on prevention with the ultimate goal of being a healthier nation. Nurses are in a role to drive this initiative and promote behavior change in the patients they encounter.
3. Recognize that patients may resist behavior change because they have misinformation or a lack of information. There are many resources available, and some are not credible. People often get advice that is not accurate from family and friends. The nurse will not know what the patient needs until he or she understands the information the patient has and where the information came from. Misinformation should be corrected, but with permission, respect, and objectivity.
4. Stay aware of public health recommendations for disease prevention and wellness care. It is important to stay informed about the behaviors that can impact our health and why. Nurses must be aware of recommended methods of prevention. Take advantage of the resources that can provide you with the necessary information to guide your practice to health promotion.

SUMMARY

Preventive care is an area that can greatly benefit from the use of motivational interviewing. Our health behaviors impact our risk for developing an acute or chronic disease, developing complications from a chronic disease, receiving an injury, and our risk of having an accident. Through behavior change we can decrease our risk for these occurrences and improve the health of our nation. Healthy People 2010 has provided us with goals for the preventive care we provide. By using motivational interviewing tactics we can successfully promote behavior change to positively impact health on individual, community, and national levels. As we head into another decade of health promotion, nurses will be taking on a greater role of promoting behavior change. We can now be armed and ready with the skills we have gained from motivational interviewing.

REFERENCES

American Academy of Family Physicians [AAFP]. (2009). Summary of recommendations for clinical preventive services, revision: 6.8. Leawood, KS: American Academy of Family Physicians.

Aspy, C., Mold, J., Thompson, D., Blondell, R., Landers, P., Reilly, K., & Wright-Eakers, L. (2008). Integrating screening and interventions for unhealthy behaviors into primary care practices. *American Journal of Preventive Medicine, 35*(5S), S373–S380.

Bastable, S. (2006). *Essentials of patient education.* Sudbury, MA: Jones and Bartlett.

Bennett, J., Lyons, K., Winters-Stone, K., Nail, L., & Scherer, J. (2007). Motivational interviewing to increase physical activity in long-term cancer survivors. *Nursing Research, 56*(1), 18–27.

Bodenheimer, T., & Handley, M. (2009). Goal-setting for behavior change in primary care: An exploration and status report. *Patient Education and Counseling, 76*(2), 174–180.

Cole, T. (2001). Smoking cessation in the hospitalized patient using the theoretical model of behavior change. *Heart & Lung, 30*(2), 148–158.

DiMarco, I., Klein, D., Clark, V., & Wilson, G. (2009). The use of motivational interviewing techniques to enhance the efficacy of guided self-help behavioral weight loss treatment. *Eating Behaviors, 10*(2), 134–136.

Flocke, S., Kelly, R., & Highland, J. (2009). Initiation of health behavior discussions during primary care outpatient visits. *Patient Education and Counseling, 75*, 214–219.

Hagan, J., Shaw, J., & Duncan, P. (2008). Bright futures: Guidelines for health supervision of infants, children and adolescents, 3rd ed. Elk Grove Village, IL: American Academy of Pediatrics.

Holtrop, J., Dosh, S., Torres, T., Arnold, A., Baumann, J., White, L., & Pathak, P. (in press). Nurse consultation support to primary care practices to increase delivery of health behavior services. *Applied Nursing Research* (in press).

Opdenacker, J., Boen, F., Coorevits, N., & Delecluse, C. (2008). Effectiveness of a lifestyle intervention and a structured exercise intervention in older adults. *Preventive Medicine, 46,* 518–524.

CHAPTER 15

Future of Motivational Interviewing in Nursing Practice

──────── **OBJECTIVES** ────────

After completing this chapter, the reader will be able to

1. Discuss the nursing profession's role in healthcare reform.
2. List at least three areas of health promotion that has been proven to be cost effective.
3. Report three suggestions for Healthy People 2020.
4. Identify three areas of research that is needed to support the effectiveness of motivational interviewing.
5. Find three resources for the nurse to participate in motivational interviewing training.

──────── **KEY TERMS** ────────

Agency for Healthcare Research and Quality
American Recovery and Reinvestment Act of 2009 (Recovery Act)
Healthy Communities Program
Motivational Interviewing Assessment: Supervisory Tools for Enhancing Proficiency

Motivational Interviewing Network of Trainers (MINT)
Training for New Trainers
U.S. Preventive Services Task Force

HEALTHCARE REFORM

In a current state of economic crisis we are forced to find cost-effective ways to decrease healthcare costs while promoting health in the United States. Nurses are on the front line and are responsible for accomplishing a majority of our goals to decrease the risk of illness and injury. Nurses are the most attainable for the patients and can provide patients with education, health promotion, health maintenance, and disease prevention skills. To improve health in the United States, we must look at our health behaviors. By changing those behaviors that lead to negative consequences, we can improve the health of patients nationwide. Motivational interviewing is a cost-effective method of promoting behavior change. These tactics can prove useful as we head into a period of healthcare reform in response to an economic crisis.

The **American Recovery and Reinvestment Act of 2009 (Recovery Act)** has been initiated. With a $1.3 trillion deficit, the government was forced to come up with a plan to rescue us from economic demise. Healthcare reform is one part of this act. A focus on health insurance is central to this movement. It is estimated that 47 million Americans are without health insurance. As more people lose their jobs due to the economy, that number is likely to increase.

The President predicts 14,000 of our population will continue to lose their health insurance coverage each day if we do not make some changes. Medicare and Medicaid costs have a significant impact on our federal deficit. The goal is to make insurance coverage available and affordable to most, if not everyone. The act seeks to decrease the out-of-pocket money needed to pay for healthcare costs, provide preventive health care, take away insurance companies' right to refuse coverage for preexisting conditions, or cancel insurance coverage due to illness (see http://www.whitehouse.gov/the_press_office/News-Conference-by-the-President-July-22-2009).

The **Agency for Healthcare Research and Quality** conducts and funds research related to healthcare costs. Among the many projects the Agency has taken on, one ongoing project is that of patient-centered care and healthcare costs. "Preliminary research suggests that patient-centered care—which is characterized by incorporating the patient's experience of illness and psychosocial context into shared physician-patient decision making—may reduce the use of healthcare services while improving health status and patient satisfaction, particularly among patients who present with unexplained, hard-to-diagnose complaints" (see http://www.ahrq.gov/news/costsfact.htm). Within this research, there are other goals (see http://www.ahrq.gov/news/costsfact.htm):

- Characterizing features of patient–physician communication that contribute to lower healthcare costs
- Identifying modifiable factors of physician interaction style that can lead to decreased use of services
- Recognition of patient emotional stress.

The provider should not be limited to physicians. Nurses, as well as other healthcare providers, can all modify how they interact and communicate with patients to improve the quality of care provided.

Chronic disease and associated costs contribute greater than 75% of all healthcare costs. Recent data state that our current national healthcare costs are approximately $2 trillion. Much of chronic disease care can be prevented by changing modifiable health behaviors. The Centers for Disease Control and Prevention has not only placed an emphasis on preventive care but also has sought to prove the cost effectiveness of preventive care. The following are examples of how preventive care can save valuable healthcare dollars in the United States (see http://www.cdc.gov/nccdphp/overview.htm):

- One dollar for water fluoridation results in $28 saved in costs for dental treatment.
- Smoking cessation programs cost an estimated $2,587 for every year a person's life is extended due to the benefits of not smoking.
- One dollar for the Safer Choice Program (school-based HIV, other sexually transmitted disease, and pregnancy prevention program) results in $2.65 saved in costs for medical care and social outcomes.
- One dollar for preconception care for women with diabetes can decrease the cost of complications in mother and baby by $5.19.
- Reaching 10,000 people with the Arthritis Self-Help Course can produce a savings of greater than $2.5 million (and decrease pain by 18% for those who participate in the course).
- Women aged 50–69 having a mammogram every 2 years results in $9,000 per year of life saved.

Clearly, we have data that demonstrate cost benefit to preventive care. Not all preventive care may save money. It is important to research specific interventions to determine costs and benefits. "Some of the measures identified by the **U.S. Preventive Services Task Force**, such as counseling adults to quit smoking, screening for colorectal cancer, and providing influenza vaccination, reduce mortality either at low cost or cost savings" (Cohen, Neumann, & Weinstein, 2008, p. 661). Many approaches can be taken to provide quality care at decreased costs. Careful evaluation of present methods, previous methods that may be superior, or creating new methods to accomplish the task of providing cost-effective treatment is important.

Efforts are being made at the community level to reduce health risk factors and support attaining health equity. The Centers for Disease Control and Prevention sponsors a program called the **Healthy Communities Program**. Through this program communities have been provided with the necessary resources to make systems and environmental changes, receive training for creating policy, and the tools to improve people's health. The inception of this program was in 2003 and continues today. Within 5 years there will be programs in over 400 communities nationwide (see http://www.cdc.gov/healthycommunitiesprogram/communities/index.htm).

HEALTHY PEOPLE 2010/2020

Healthy People is not an initiative that has run its course. This is a program that will continue because it helps guide our practice and is designed to improve health in the United States. It is not possible to be a country without illness or injury. There will always be room for improvement in our practice. Our practice is not limited to the individuals that we encounter but includes communities and, on a larger scale, our nation. In previous chapters we looked at the goals and objectives of Healthy People 2010. As we head into a new decade, the future of a healthy nation will be addressed in Healthy People 2020.

At the time of this writing the goals have yet to be established for Healthy People 2020. There is a consortium that invites agencies and organizations to help develop and integrate the goals into their programs and use the goals to create new healthcare programs (see http://www.healthypeople.gov/hp2020/Consortium/Default.aspx). Currently, many dedicated groups have made a commitment to the Healthy People 2020 initiative. As we move forward, the scientific-based goals and objectives will allow us to continue with evidence-based nursing practices.

There have been thirteen meetings of the Secretary's Advisory Committee on National Health Promotion and Disease Prevention Objectives for 2020. The most recent information available is from the eighth meeting in January 2009. During this meeting there was discussion about the current economic crisis of our nation and the relationship between health and productivity. A healthier nation will be more productive in the workforce and improve our economic status. The U.S. Department of Health and Human Services was developing specific objectives with baseline and target data. There was discussion about making the information user friendly to increase involvement in achieving the goals established. The Task Force on Community Preventive Services had developed 210 recommendations and a list of 25 top priority areas. It was determined that a tool could potentially be offered to help with cost analysis.

Evaluating cost effectiveness can be very difficult, and there is debate about how to increase the amount of data available and ensure that it is accurate. One challenge is conducting necessary research to support the development and continuation of Healthy People 2020. Research is costly, and the economic state of our nation does not support the research that is needed. To be successful with Healthy People 2020, there are committee members that are dedicated to reviewing Healthy People 2000 and Healthy People 2010 to determine what was effective and what was ineffective. All this information is helping to shape this next initiative (see http://www.healthypeople.gov/hp2020/advisory/FACA8MinutesDay1.htm).

On the second day of this meeting, there was discussion about the difficulties that communities and state programs are having due to budget cuts. With this in mind, the following suggestions were made for Healthy People 2020 (see http://www.healthypeople.gov/hp2020/advisory/FACA8minutesDay2.htm):

- Success should be judged by the extent to which it measurably improves the health of the nation.
- Healthy People should do fewer things but do them well.
- Targets should be measurable, realistic, and achievable.
- If it can't be measured, don't make it a target.
- Continuous quality improvement is critically important through frequent, periodic measurement.

By the end of the meeting, there was the suggestion to prepare information to be submitted to the U.S. Department of Health and Human Services, as this is the governing body and must accept all proposals set forth in Healthy People 2020.

Public meetings will be held in October and November 2009. The goal of these meetings is to receive input from the public for objectives and topic areas for Healthy People 2020. Information will also be provided about the framework, topic areas, and an overview of the potential objectives (see http://www.healthy people.gov/hp2020/regional/2009agenda.asp).

Public comment was sought to help those who are creating Healthy People 2020. Areas open to comment were as follows (see http://www.healthypeople. gov/hp2020/Comments/SubjectFocus.aspx):

- Vision, mission, overarching goals
- Conceptual approach/organizing framework
- Users and implementation
- Other issues/general comments
- 2010 focus areas and objectives

The following overarching goals that were open for comment were as follows (see http://www.healthypeople.gov/hp2020/Comments/SubjectFocus.aspx):

- Achieve health equity, eliminate disparities, and improve health for all groups
- Eliminate preventable disease, disability, injury, and premature death
- Create social and physical environments that promote good health for all
- Promote healthy development and healthy behaviors across every stage of life.

MOTIVATIONAL INTERVIEWING AND NURSING: MOVING TOWARD THE FUTURE

Understanding where we have been and where we are heading is important. We have a responsibility as individuals and nurses to improve the health of our nation, one patient at a time. Just as they say in commercials for Gardisil, "one less." If we can prevent one less risk factor for each patient we encounter, we can change the world. During a time of economic crisis there is a need to promote and maintain health and prevent accidents, injuries, disease, and complications of disease in a cost-effective manner. This may seem impossible, but nurses have seen the impossible become possible. Nursing has progressed from a role of following orders to a role of guiding healthcare practice. We have gone from telling our patients to involving our patients in making healthcare decisions. We have gone from reading books to writing books. We have gone from gaining insight from research to conducting research. Nothing is impossible.

We have a driving force from the Healthy People initiative. We have tools to accomplish the goals set before us. We have a responsibility to provide scientific-based, cost-effective care. We have the nation's health in our hands. Motivational interviewing is a significant tool we have available. It is cost effective and can be used in almost every situation. Research has continued to prove its effectiveness in areas of alcohol and drug addiction, exercise, smoking cessation, asthma, and diabetes management. As we move forward, nurses have an opportunity to evaluate the effectiveness of motivational interviewing in other areas as we accomplish current Healthy People goals.

Some see the nurse as the actual tool for change. "Our task is to become tools for change, getting to know the patient first in order to help him or her resolve ambivalence and become motivated to change" (Roberts, 2009, p. 8). Nurses have used methods of therapeutic communication throughout the profession. Motivational interviewing is basically another therapeutic method of communication. By using motivational interviewing tactics, we become a tool for the patient's health behavior change. We have the ability to unlock the doors of resistance, balance the scale of ambivalence, and mobilize change talk to action.

I see motivational interviewing as a set of communication tools that nurses can have available at all times and that can help them be prepared for most situations. The nurse has a vital role in helping patients achieve optimal health and self-actualization. We cannot do this alone. We need to have many tools to accomplish our goals. Motivational interviewing can be used with people from every age group, ethnic background, socioeconomic status, and religious stance. It is valuable in every environment in which the nurse may practice. And it can promote behavior change for those who are ready to change, ambivalent about change, or resistant to change. No other tool can be so broadly used and be effective across the population.

RESEARCH NEEDS

More research is needed to prove the value of motivational interviewing in health care and nursing practice. Economics impacts every area of nursing practice. As we face the current economic crisis, it is important to evaluate the cost effectiveness of motivational interviewing. Although some studies have been done, there is a need to seek evidence of costs and benefits to promoting behavior change to improve health, decreasing risk factors for disease and injury, and supporting self-management. Motivational interviewing is designed to accomplish each of these tasks.

Throughout this text we discussed the use of motivational interviewing in various areas of health care. What research has been done is limited. Those studies that have proved effectiveness of this technique have done so in few areas. The outcome is that we are pushing the envelope and assuming this is effective in areas that have not yet been studied. There is an assumption that it is possible to transfer the knowledge we gain in one area to another area with the same results. This is not uncommon in health care. If there is a possibility that a communication technique may be useful in different situations, it is reasonable to explore the possibilities. This is what drives research to ensure we continue to provide evidence-based practice.

The areas of needed research regarding motivational interviewing and nursing practice are vast. The more we learn and the more we practice with motivational interviewing techniques, the more we will find that we need to know. Although not all inclusive, the following are some potential research questions that still need to be answered:

- What are the costs involved in using motivational interviewing to promote behavior change? (This would include costs of training, costs of performing the task, and cost benefit of the particular behavior change.)
- What is the impact of using motivational interviewing on quality of care provided?
- What is the best way to ensure nurses are trained adequately to provide care with motivational interviewing skills? (Is it face to face training, internet training, or self-educating? How can we address each learner's needs?)
- How does the nurse's level of self-awareness affect the success of using motivational interviewing to promote behavior change? (Are nurses who have strong self-awareness more effective at using motivational interviewing?)
- Does using motivational interviewing in nursing practice increase career satisfaction or decrease burn-out in nursing?
- What is the nurse's contribution to increasing the patient's feelings of empowerment? (Was there an action or words the nurse shared that triggered a sense of empowerment? And if so, what were they?)
- Do the nurse and patient agree on a point in the conversation where the patient found clarity and started the path toward change? (Do the patient and nurse have the same perspective on a pivotal moment in the encounter?)
- What are the barriers to incorporating motivational interviewing into nursing practice? (Are these barriers personal, system wide, or educational opportunities?)

MOTIVATIONAL INTERVIEWING TRAINING

Motivational interviewing is a skill set that must be learned, practiced, revisited for further education needs or advanced training, and continued to learn the many tactics that make this a valuable tool in promoting behavior change. It is not a simple task to be followed. It requires self-exploration and self-awareness. These are not simple tasks that can be quickly learned but rather are shaped over a period of time. As we become comfortable in using the tools of motivational interviewing, we become more adventurous and less inhibited in our exploration of ourselves and our patients. What we learn about ourselves will impact the way we communicate with our patients. Each interaction shapes the next as we see what is working and what is not. We become more accepting of our role to help the patient become empowered to make their own healthcare choices. We let go of the need to determine what is best for someone else and the need to fix everything that may be broken in another person's life. We learn to respect that each patient is unique and may not want to make a change.

William Miller and Theresa Moyers identified eight stages in learning motivational interviewing (Madson, Loignon, & Lane, 2009; see http://www.motivationalinterview.org/TNT_Manual_Nov_08.pdf):

1. Overall spirit of motivational interviewing: Understand the underlying philosophy of motivational interviewing that "is composed of three major tenets: collaboration, evocation, and autonomy" (Madson et al., 2009, p. 102).
2. OARS: client-centered counseling skills: "Counselors are encouraged to be proficient in their ability to use open questions, affirm the client's responses, apply accurate reflections, and provide summaries when necessary" (Madson et al., 2009, p. 102).
3. Recognizing change talk and resistance—DARN: Desire, Ability, Reasons, and Need for change: Identify change talk, commitment to behavior change language, and signs of resistance.
4. Eliciting and strengthening change talk: Evoking and reinforcing change talk and commitment language; using OARS skills appropriately.
5. Rolling with resistance: "In this stage, individuals are encouraged to view resistive behavior not as pathological or defensive but as a natural component of the change process" (Madson et al., 2009, p. 102). Resistance can be a positive factor in promoting behavior change.
6. Developing a change plan: Properly using timing and negotiation skills to recognize when the patient is ready to change and help the patient through the change process.
7. Consolidating commitment: Moving the patient from "I think I can" to "I will"; helping the patient increase the strength of their commitment to change.

8. Transition and blending: Using motivational interviewing along with other techniques without losing the philosophy or effectiveness of motivational interviewing.

A sample outline for basic motivational interviewing training is provided in **Motivational Interviewing Assessment: Supervisory Tools for Enhancing Proficiency** (Table 15-1). Once this initial training is complete, the nurse must put it into practice. This allows time and experience necessary for growth. "Trainee self-confidence is an important factor relating to one probability of engaging in a behavior . . . an individual is more likely to engage in a behavior if they are confident in their abilities to perform the behavior" (Madson et al., 2009, p. 107). Increased use of the skills will increase comfort level and self-confidence in using motivational interviewing in nursing practice.

Research has shown that participating in motivational interviewing training sessions do not provide sufficient preparation to be proficient. "Ongoing feedback and mentoring were needed in order for most counselors to use MI skillfully" (Martino et al., 2006, p. 7). This feedback can be obtained through evaluation of tape recordings of nurse–patient conversations. Use of Motivational Interviewing Skill Code and Motivational Interviewing Treatment Integrity will help to not only determine the effectiveness of the communication, but can offer the nurse important feedback that can help shape future practice (see Chapter 3). This allows us to see what is working within our interactions that move our patients closer to behavior change, when appropriate. It also allows us to learn from our mistakes and ultimately, improve the effectiveness of our practice.

There are different levels of training. There is a **Motivational Interviewing Network of Trainers (MINT)** that consists of trainers worldwide. These trainers are motivational interviewing experts and have advanced skills in motivational interviewing that provides them the ability to train other trainers and offer advanced training to novices. Training sessions they offer can be located on their Web site (see http://www.motivationalinterview.org). (See Figure 15-1 for recommended advancement through trainings.) Titles of some of their current training sessions available are as follows (see http://motivationalinterview.org/training/index.html#training):

- Introduction to Motivational Interviewing
- Advanced Motivational Interviewing
- Supervisor Motivational Interviewing
- Motivational Interviewing and Health Behavior Change
- Motivational Interviewing with Trauma Related Issues
- Motivational Interviewing in Group Treatment: Theory and Skill Building Practice
- MI Coding 3.0 and Skill Coaching

Table 15-1.   Sample Syllabus for a Basic Motivational Interviewing Training Workshop

1. Motivational Interviewing as a Style and Spirit
   a. Person-centered versus disorder-centered approach
   b. Motivation as a state or stage, not a fixed character trait
   c. Client defensiveness or resistance as a therapeutic process
   d. Effect of therapist style on client behavior
   e. Collaboration, not confrontation
   f. Resistance and change talk: opposite sides of ambivalence
   g. Respect for client autonomy and choice
2. Underlying Principles of Motivational Interviewing
   a. Express empathy
   b. Develop discrepancy
   c. Roll with resistance, avoiding argumentation
   d. Support self-efficacy
3. Stages of Change
   a. Precontemplation
   b. Contemplation
   c. Preparation
   d. Action
   e. Maintenance
   f. Relapse
4. Motivational Interviewing Micro-Skills: OARS
   a. Open-ended questions
   b. Affirmations
   c. Reflective listening
   d. Summaries
5. OARS Practice, Especially in Forming Reflections
   a. Types of reflections
      i. Simple
      ii. Amplified
      iii. Double-sided
   b. Levels of reflection
      i. Repeat
      ii. Rephrase
      iii. Paraphrase
6. Exploring Ambivalence
   a. Decision balance
   b. Developing discrepancy

      i. Exploring goals and values

      ii. Looking forward

7. Role of and Rolling With Resistance

  a. What does it look and feel like?

      i. Arguing

      ii. Interrupting

      iii. Negating or "denial"

      iv. Ignoring

  b. What is it?

      i. A cue to change strategies

      ii. A normal reaction to having freedoms decreased or denied

      iii. An interpersonal process

  c. Ways to roll

      i. Reflections

      ii. Shift focus

      iii. Reframe

      iv. Agreement with a twist

      v. Emphasize personal choice and control

      vi. Coming alongside

8. Concept of Readiness: Importance + Confidence

  a. As related to stages of change

  b. Methods of measuring

      i. Readiness ruler

      ii. Instruments like URICA and SOCRATES

9. Change Talk

  a. Recognizing DARN C statements

      i. Desire

      ii. Ability

      iii. Reasons

      iv. Needs

      v. Commitment level

  b. Eliciting change talk

      i. Evocative questions

      ii. Elaborations

10. Developing a Change Plan

  a. Role of information and advice

  b. Menu options

  c. Asking for commitment

Source: From Martino et al. (2006).

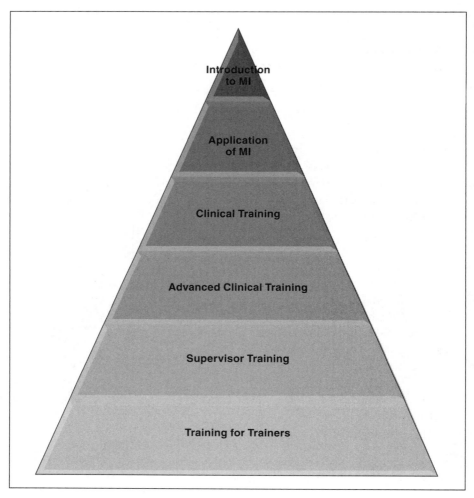

Figure 15-1.   Progression Through Motivational Interviewing (MI) Training

Source: http://www.motivationalinterview.org/TNT_Manual_Nov_08.pdf

This is just a sample of training that is available through this network of train-ers. Access to training videos is also available through MINT.

Different goals can be accomplished with different levels of training. The MINT has made resources available for trainers. It is entitled Motivational In-terviewing: **Training for New Trainers.** Within this resource guide they offer recommendations for training levels and goals that can be accomplished within each level. The first level of training that introduces motivational interviewing strives for the following goals (see http://www.motivationalinterview.org/TNT_Manual_Nov_08.pdf):

- To experience the basics of motivational interviewing and decide level of interest in learning more
- To be familiar with the fundamental spirit and principles of motivational interviewing
- To be acquainted with relevant evidence of efficacy
- To directly experience the motivational interviewing approach and contrast it with others.

Goals for the application of motivational interviewing are as follows (see http://www.motivationalinterview.org/TNT_Manual_Nov_08.pdf):

- To learn one or more specific applications of motivational interviewing
- To be acquainted with the fundamental spirit of motivational interviewing
- To learn practical guidelines for a specific application within the spirit of motivational interviewing
- To have direct practice in and experience of this particular application
- To decide level of interest in learning more.

Clinical training is the next level of motivational interviewing training. Goals for this level of training are as follows (see http://www.motivationalinterview.org/TNT_Manual_Nov_08.pdf):

- To learn the basic clinical style of motivational interviewing and how to continue learning it in practice
- To understand the fundamental spirit and principles of motivational interviewing
- To strengthen empathic counseling skills (OARS)
- To understand and practice the directive aspects of motivational interviewing
- To experience and practice a motivational interviewing style for meeting resistance
- To learn the fundamental client language cues (change talk and resistance) that allow continued feedback and learning in practice.

Advanced clinical training offers the following abilities (see http://www.motivationalinterview.org/TNT_Manual_Nov_08.pdf):

- To move from basic competence to more advanced clinical skillfulness in motivational interviewing
- To have intensive observed practice in advanced motivational interviewing skills

- To receive individual feedback regarding motivational interviewing practice
- To update knowledge of motivational interviewing (recent research and development).

The fifth level of motivational interviewing training is supervisor training. Goals set for this level of training are as follows (see http://www.motivational interview.org/TNT_Manual_Nov_08.pdf):

- To be prepared to guide an ongoing group in learning motivational interviewing
- To understand the sequence of skills for acquiring motivational interviewing proficiency
- To learn observational/analytic methods for evaluating motivational interviewing
- To learn methods for facilitating practice improvement over time
- To be prepared to certify motivational interviewing practitioners and maintain quality control.

The sixth and final level of training is the training for the trainers. The following goals have been set for this level of training (see http://www.motivational interview.org/TNT_Manual_Nov_08.pdf):

- To learn a flexible range of skills and methods for helping others learn motivational interviewing
- To learn and practice an array of motivational interviewing training methods
- To enhance confidence in training and demonstrating motivational interviewing
- To assess the specific needs and context of trainees and to design and adapt training approaches accordingly
- To update knowledge of motivational interviewing and training (recent research/developments)
- To participate in the international motivational interviewing network of trainers.

The skills we gain through training will only enhance our ability to promote health, support health maintenance, promote healthy behavior change, and prevent accidents, injuries, and complications of chronic illness. These, in addition to the other skills nurses possess, will allow us to fulfill our role as change agent to promote a healthier nation.

RESOURCES FOR MOTIVATIONAL INTERVIEWING TRAINING

There are many methods of training available. It is recommended that any training involve some role playing or practice opportunities. Didactic learning provides a basis for our motivational interviewing training but is not as successful when used alone. Initial training should be obtained from a reputable source. Ongoing training can occur in face-to-face sessions, review tapes of interactions, and "webinars." The one single important source of feedback on our motivational interviewing skills is the patient with whom we interact. Immediate feedback is available. We will know if we are offering accurate reflections, recognizing ambivalence, and change talk. "Once you learn to differentiate the signals of change talk and resistance statements from the background of client speech, you have the cues you need both to work more effectively with each person and to learn from each person" (Miller & Rollnick, 2002, p. 181).

The following is a listing of some valuable training resources:

- MINT: list of trainers and training opportunities
- Kaiser Permanente
- The Institute of Motivation and Change
- Jeff Allison Training
- Stephenrollnick.com
- Training videos:
- Motivational Interviewing (Brief Therapy for Addictions Video Series)
  ○ Motivational Interviewing Training Video: A Tool for Learners
  ○ MI Training DVDs: Focusing on Importance, Confidence and Readiness
  ○ MI in Practice: The Edinburgh Interview 2006
  ○ Engaging Motivation
  ○ Motivational Interviewing: Professional Training Series

SUMMARY

The United States is a nation of many resources. Currently, we are in a state of economic crisis. This lends to an increased need for health promotion and cost-effective methods to promote behavior change to improve the health of our nation. The nursing profession has a responsibility to our patients, our communities, and our nation to promote health, decrease health risks, and prevent illness and injury. Healthy People 2010 and Healthy People 2020 are strong driving forces that provide us with guidelines to promote the health of our nation. Motivational interviewing is a unique set of communication skills and tactics to promote behavior change to achieve a higher level of health. With proper training, we can become proficient in these skills. Although research supports the effectiveness of motivational interviewing, more research is needed. As we take steps into the future, nursing as a profession will be essential to the achievement of the Healthy People goals. And we will become a healthier nation.

REFERENCES

Cohen, J., Neumann, P., & Weinstein, M. (2008). Does preventive care save money? Health economics and the presidential candidates. *New England Journal of Medicine, 358*(7), 661–663.

Madson, M., Loignon, A., & Lane, C. (2009). Training in motivational interviewing: A systematic review. *Journal of Substance Abuse Treatment, 36*(1), 101–109.

Martino, S., Ball, S. A., Gallon, S. L., Hall, D., Garcia, M., Ceperich, S., Farentinos, C., Hamilton, J., & Hausotter, W. (2006). *Motivational interviewing assessment: Supervisory tools for enhancing proficiency.* Salem, OR: Northwest Frontier Addiction Technology Transfer Center, Oregon Health and Science University.

Miller, W., & Rollnick, S. (2002). *Motivational interviewing: Preparing people for change* (2nd ed.). New York: The Guilford Press.

Roberts, D. (2009). Becoming a tool for change. *MEDSURG Nursing, 18*(1), 8.

Index

Page numbers followed by *f* or *t* indicate figures or tables, respectively.